Hollow Earth Messengers

ARE TAKING THE AGE PILL

DUSTIN LEE DEN HOOD

ACKNOWLEDGMENTS

To Jim, my mentor, and Billie Faye Woodard, both are extremely nice and kind Genuine people, but I think Jim is just more loud, I guess you might put it.

CONTENTS

INTRODUCTION

IT IS NATURAL for us to get sick. When the weather changes drastically, some of us experience headaches, cough and colds. We can determine the causes of the illness and apply solutions. But before consulting the doctor or even popping a pill for relief, here is a wonder medicine for all kinds of illness. An easy, no side-effect, way of being well is through quantum healing.

This popular healing technique is currently used around the world but only a few understand what it truly means. According to Merriam-Webster dictionary, quantum is "any of the very small increments or parcels into which many forms of energy are subdivided". If we relate it to our physical body, quantum is simply equivalent to our cells. The cells are also known as the building blocks of our body. And these small units of life are often the most ignored factor when we are finding ways to get well.

In order to be healthy, it is important that you start healing the cells. You should first look at the changes within your body that causes the illness before you direct your attention to external factors. This can only be done if you listen to what your body is telling you. Analyze your thoughts, emotions, feelings and energy. Notice how these internal factors affect your body and your surroundings. Quantum healing involves both the mind and body.

It is important to remember that all internal factors have corresponding effects to the body. Dr. Deepak Chopra even stated, "Your body is just the place your memory calls home." Positive experiences stores good memories in the cells. In turn, the cells function well and positive energy flows naturally to new cells. However, negative experiences will only store bad memories in the cells. The contained negative energy will be trapped in the cells and will block the positive flow of energy. This buildup of negative energy will cause discomfort manifested as pain or other types of illness.

Sometimes your body needs assistance to remove toxins, strengthen the immune system, or to provide trace elements that are hard to source in our diet. It can be difficult sometimes to find reliable, high quality sources of natural help. With this knowledge, my body is healthier today than ever before.

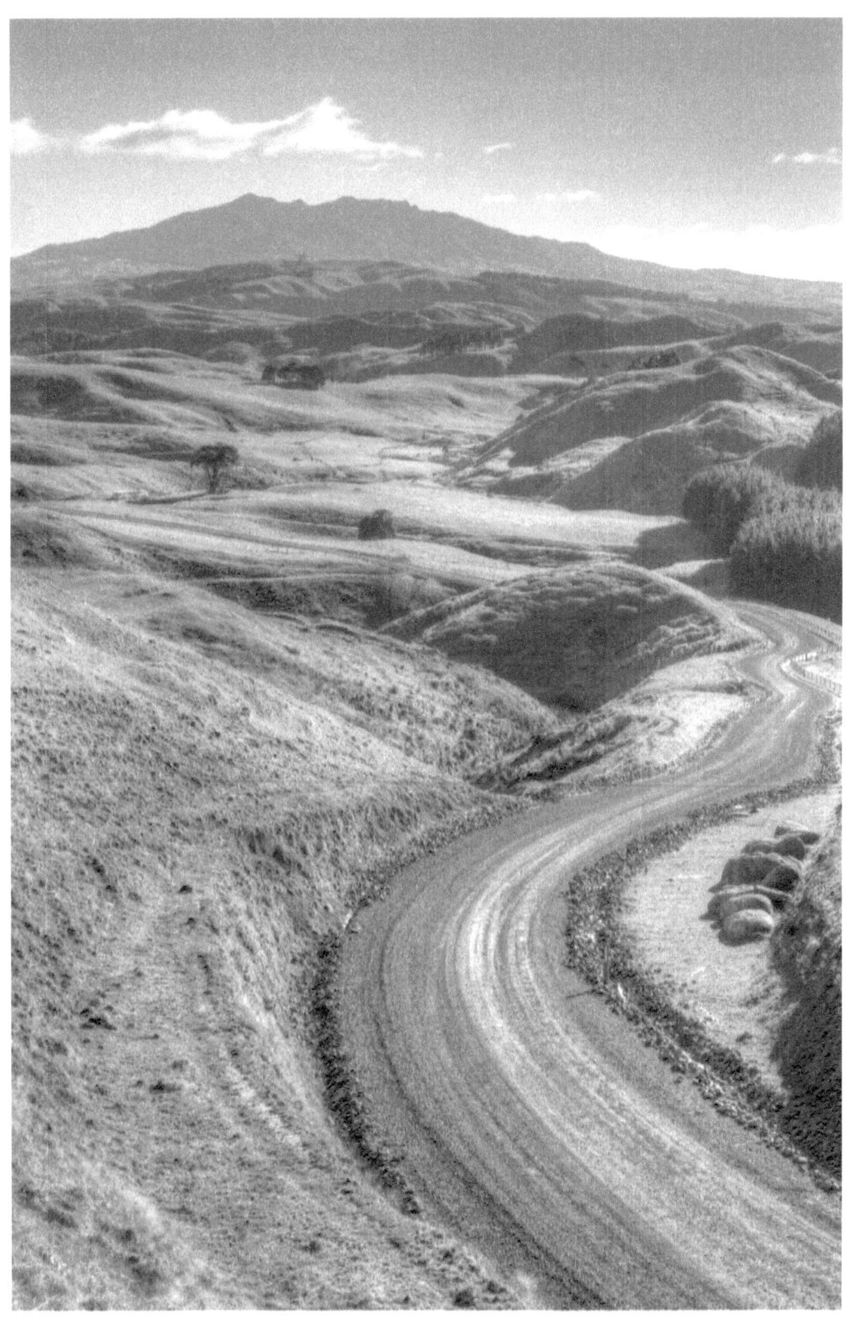

THE HOLLOW EARTH

THE HOLLOW EARTH is a pseudoscientific concept proposing that the planet Earth is entirely Hollow or contains a substantial interior space. The scientific community has dismissed the notion since at least the late-18th century. The concept of a Hollow Earth occurs many times in folklore and as the premise for subterranean fiction, and a subgenre of adventure fiction. It is also featured in some present day pseudoscientific and conspiracy theories.

Concave Hollow Earths

An example of a concave Hollow Earth. Humans live on the interior, with the universe in the center. Instead of saying that humans live on the outside surface of a hollow planet sometimes called a "convex" Hollow Earth hypothesis some have claimed humans live on the inside surface of a Hollow spherical world, so that our universe itself lies in that world's interior. This has been called the "concave" Hollow Earth hypothesis or skycentrism.

Cyrus Teed, a doctor from upstate New York, proposed such a concave Hollow Earth in 1869, calling his scheme "Cellular Cosmogony". Teed founded a group called the Koreshan Unity based on this notion, which he called Koreshanity. The main colony survives as a preserved Florida state historic site, at Estero, Florida, but all of Teed's followers have now died. Teed's followers claimed to have experimentally verified the concavity of the Earth's curvature, through surveys of the Florida coastline making use of "rectilineator" equipment.

Several twentieth-century German writers, including Peter Bender, Johannes Lang, Karl Neupert, and Fritz Braut, published works advocating the Hollow Earth hypothesis, or Hohlweltlehre. It has even been reported, although apparently without historical documentation, that Adolf Hitler was influenced by concave Hollow Earth ideas and sent an expedition in an unsuccessful attempt to spy on the British fleet by pointing infrared cameras up at the sky.

The Egyptian mathematician Mostafa Abdelkader wrote several scholarly papers working out a detailed mapping of the Concave Earth model.

According to Gardner, this hypothesis posits that light rays travel in circular paths, and slow as they approach the center of the spherical star-filled cavern. No energy can reach the center of the cavern, which corresponds to no point a finite distance away from Earth in the widely accepted scientific cosmology. A drill, Gardner says, would lengthen as it traveled away from the cavern and eventually pass through the "point at infinity" corresponding to the center of the Earth in the widely accepted scientific cosmology. Supposedly no experiment can distinguish between the two cosmologies.

Gardner notes that "most mathematicians believe that an inside-out universe, with properly adjusted physical laws, is empirically irrefutable". Gardner rejects the concave Hollow Earth hypothesis on the basis of Occam's razor.

Purportedly verifiable hypotheses of a "Concave Hollow Earth" need to be distinguished from a thought experiment which defines a coordinate transformation such that the interior of the Earth becomes "exterior" and the exterior becomes "interior". (For example, in spherical coordinates, let radius r go to R2/r where R is the Earth's radius.) The transformation entails corresponding changes to the forms of physical laws. This is not a hypothesis but an illustration of the fact that any description of the physical world can be equivalently expressed in more than one way.

Seismic

The picture of the structure of the Earth that has been arrived at through the study of seismic waves is quite different from the Hollow Earth hypothesis. The time it takes for seismic waves to travel through and around the Earth directly contradicts a hollow sphere. The evidence indicates that the Earth is filled with solid rock (mantle and crust), liquid nickel-iron alloy (outer core), and solid nickel-iron (inner core).

Gravity

Another set of scientific arguments against a Hollow Earth or any hollow planet comes from gravity. Massive objects tend to clump together gravitationally, creating non-hollow spherical objects such as stars and planets. The solid sphere is the best way in which to minimize the gravitational potential energy of a physical object; having hollowness is unfavorable in the energetic sense. In addition, ordinary matter is not strong enough to support a hollow shape of planetary size against the force of gravity; a planet-sized hollow shell with the known, observed thickness of the Earth's crust would not be able to achieve hydrostatic equilibrium with its own mass and would collapse.

Density

Based upon the size of the Earth and the force of gravity on its surface, the average density of the planet Earth is 5.515 g/cm3, and typical densities of surface rocks are only half that (about 2.75 g/cm3). If any significant portion of the Earth were hollow, the average density would be much lower than that of surface rocks. The only way for Earth to have the force of gravity that it does is for much more dense material to make up a large part of the interior. Nickel-iron alloy under the conditions expected in a non-Hollow Earth would have densities ranging from about 10 to 13 g/cm3, which brings the average density of Earth to its observed value.

Direct observation

Drilling holes does not provide direct evidence against the hypothesis. The deepest hole drilled to date is the Kola Superdeep Borehole, with a true vertical drill-depth of more than 7.5 miles (12 kilometers). However, the distance to the center of the Earth is nearly 4,000 miles (6,400 kilometers). Oil wells with longer depths are not vertical wells; the total depths quoted are measured depth (MD) or equivalently, along-hole depth (AHD) as these wells are deviated to horizontal.

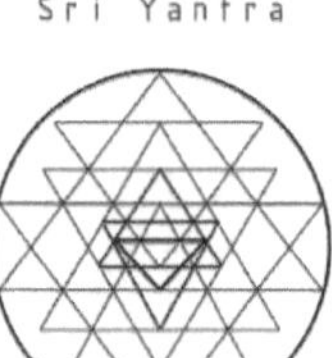

Sri Yantra

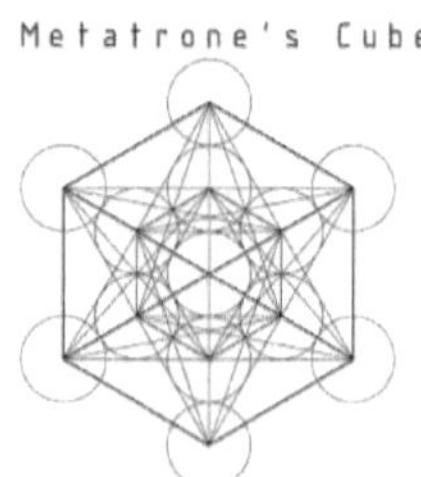

Metatrone's Cube

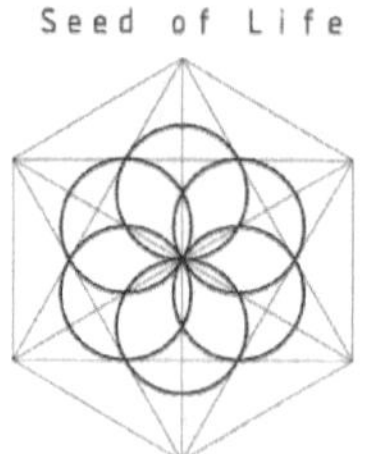

Seed of Life

SACRED GEOMETRY GREAT BUNDLE

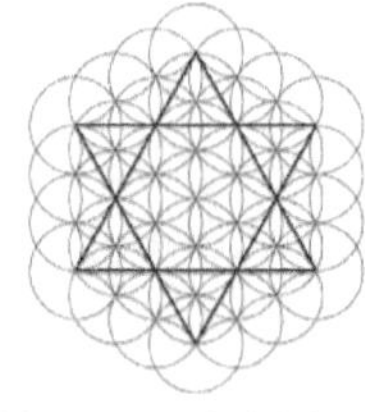

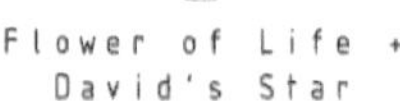

Flower of Life +
David's Star

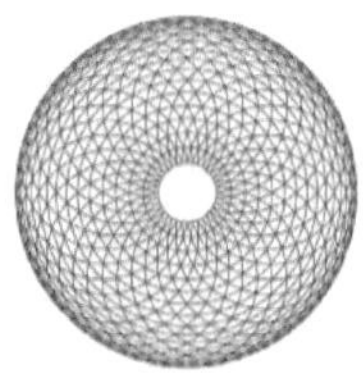

Torus yantra
(Hypnotic Eye)

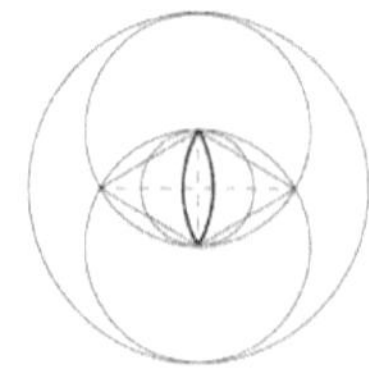

Vesica Piscis

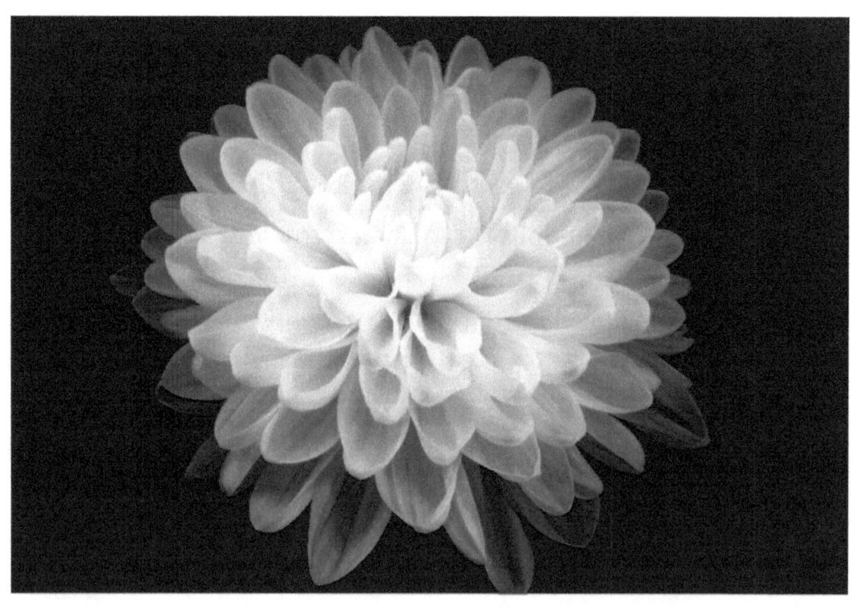

THE SCIENTIFIC BASIS FOR HOLLOW EARTH

POSSIBLY THE FIRST PERSON to scientifically speculate about a Hollow Earth was none other than Edmund Halley, of Halley's Comet fame. Proposed in 1692 as a way of explaining anomalous compass readings, Halley's theory is that the planet is a series of nested, spherical shells, spinning in different directions, all surrounding a central core. In his estimation, based on readings of the magnetic field and what he knew of the gravitational pull of the sun and the moon on the Earth, this model could account for any inaccuracies in his readings of the magnetic fields of the planet. He also posited that the space between each shell may have had luminous atmospheres capable of supporting life.

Halley's strange idea was expanded upon over the next few centuries, tossing out the messy view of multiple spheres for the much funner vision that the entire interior of the Earth is just one, impossibly large cavern. Generally, this new view of the Hollow Earth is accompanied with the theory of a small sun that hangs in the very center, creating a lush, livable environment on the flip side of the Earth's surface. According to a number of Hollow Earth websites, this vision was developed among famous mathematicians and scientists such as Leonhard Euler in the 18th century and Sir John Leslie in the 19th century, although the sources for these accreditations seem to be somewhat nebulous.

Regardless of where it originated, the model of a Hollow Earth managed to grow and survive. In 1818, John Cleves Symmes, Jr. published his Circular No. 1, declaring to the world that the Earth is Hollow. Symmes, a veteran of the War of 1812 and unsuccessful trader, soon became maybe the most famous and successful proponent of the Hollow Earth theory. His initial vision of the Earth's interior was like a simplified version of Halley's multi-layered model, with the exception that Symmes' version included huge holes at the North and South poles which allowed access to the hidden world inside. These holes, his unique addition to Hollow Earth theory, would even come to be known as "Symmes Holes."

In his very first declaration, Symmes proposed to mount an expedition to the North Pole, where he was sure they could locate one of these apertures, and gain access to the inner Earth. He too believed that the interior of the Earth, not only could, but did support life, saying in Circular No. 1, that the inside of the Earth would be "stocked with thrifty vegetables and animals if not men." Symmes believed that his theory was not science fiction, but science fact, and that it applied not only to the Earth but too all planetary bodies. To him, the whole universe was hollow.

Even in the 19th century, Symmes' theories were greeted with derision from the public and scientific community, but he would not be silenced. Symmes continued to campaign, giving lectures and publishing letters about the Hollow Earth, always angling for an expedition to the North Pole that would prove his theory. Barrelling right through the skeptics, Symmes was eventually able to convince enough people of the possibility of his Hollow Earth that, in 1822, he and his supporters actually got Congress to vote on funding for his expedition. The grant was shot down, but Symmes' belief in the Inner Earth never died. He continued to campaign for the theory until his death in 1849.

Even after Symmes' death his idea continued to thrive amongst believers. Students and admirers of Symmes' work, and even Symmes' own son continued to publish materials explaining the increasingly odd theory.

One bizarre offshoot of the traditional Hollow Earth theory, put forth by natural healer and eventual cult leader, Cyrus Teed, even inverted the idea, devising a "cellular cosmology" that placed the entire universe inside a shell. According to Teed's thinking, we were actually living on the inside of the Hollow Earth, looking up at the universe, which itself was just an illusion created by a strange solar mechanism. The stars were just reflections of the mechanism's light. Teed's theory managed to gain enough traction that a small cult developed around him, called the Koreshan Unity after Teed renamed himself Koresh. The Koreshans established an extensive colony in Estero, Florida in 1894, but most of the community disbanded after Teed's death in 1908.

Both Teed and Symmes still have monuments dedicated to their work and beliefs. The location where the Koreshan community made their home is now protected as the Koreshan State Historic Site, while Ohio's Hollow Earth Monument is dedicated to Symmes' work.

Even as unbelievable as the beliefs of Symmes and Teed were, as the Hollow Earth theory grew into the 20th century, it began to take on an even more supernatural air.

From Science to Science Fiction

In 1864 Jules Verne published A Journey to the Centre of the Earth, which proposed a weird world inside our own, and while it was not the first work of fiction to propose such a thing (it could be argued that the first such work of fiction regarding the weird world inside of our own is Dante's poem, Inferno), Verne's work quickly became the benchmark for such fantasy tales, giving steam to a whole sub-genre of subterranean science-fiction. Many of these stories used the theories of Halley and Symmes as jumping off points for tales of weird prehistoric jungles and highly advanced lost races of humans. The 1892 novel, The Goddess of Atvatabar, or The History of the Discovery of the Interior World, used Symmes' model as a basis for a tale of a rich interior world inhabited by a race of spiritually enlightened beings. This vision of the Hollow Earth would seem to be one of the prime inspirations of many of the current tropes among modern Hollow Earth theory.

Modern belief in the Hollow Earth theory can be a bit hard to pin down, encompassing such disparate subjects as the Northern Lights and even an escaping Hitler ("The Germans did make it to Hollow Earth. They made a deal with the people in the Hollow Earth."). The largest proponents of the theory seem to be singular thinkers like Cluff, who often have their own spin on the hypothesis, or hold up what they consider to be the true evidence. Despite the variations, a few themes do seem to be common among Hollow Earth truthers.

Among most believers, the inside of the Hollow Earth is a lush tropical paradise that very likely houses an advanced race of humans/aliens/giants. In most scenarios, the inhabitants are the descendants of ancient races such as the Lemurians or, as in Cluff's view, the Lost Ten Tribes of Israel, guided there through the North polar opening by God himself. No matter where they come from, they are generally characterized as peace-loving, and advanced far beyond our own. "They have flying saucer technology. They live lives of perfect health for hundreds of years.

The perfect climate believed to exist in the Hollow Earth is said to produce animals and people that are larger and far healthier than those on the surface. "It has a perfect temperature. God made the inner sun so that it provides heat, during the night, and a little bit less at night. Trees grow up to a thousand feet tall. Humans even grow up to 15 feet tall," Cluff told us. "Because of the ideal conditions, animal life grows really large also." This inner world is sometimes called or associated with Agartha, a legendary city at the Earth's core often tied to Eastern mysticism.

Fear of a Hollow Planet

If it is to be believed that the Earth is in fact hollow, and home to all manner of super-race and megafauna, why have we never contacted them, or gone there? According to Cluff, we have, but an international banking conspiracy has worked to cover up the existence of the Hollow Earth, and hide evidence of any Symmes Holes. This sort of paranoid, conspiratorial thinking tends to be another hallmark among modern Hollow Earth believers, because, really there is no other force that could be keeping us from engaging with the wonders of the Inner Earth, given our current level of technology and exploratory freedom.

One of the most popular pieces of evidence for Hollow Earth is a supposed secret journal entry by Admiral Richard Byrd, who claimed to be the first person to fly over the North and South pole. According to believers, Byrd's secret journal from 1947 included a report of flying into one of the Symmes Holes, and making contact with the race that lives inside the Earth.

Through the mid-2000s and into the early 2010s, Cluff was actually a part of a long-gestating expedition known most recently as the North Pole Inner Earth Expedition. Unfortunately, after a number of setbacks including backers and members of the team falling victim to calamities ranging from cancer to fatal plane crashes, the expedition was put on hiatus. Had the expedition been successful, the team would have chartered one of the world's largest ice breaking ships straight to the North Pole, where they would have attempted to contact the denizens of the Hollow Earth through the hole they believed they would find. Cluff believes that the various setbacks to the project are the work of the international banking conspiracy, but is hopeful that they will someday be able to get funding, and a new expedition leader to help continue the project. And even if he doesn't, the Hollow Earth theory will likely continue on. Until humans can actually peer into the Earth's core, who can say that it's not filled with Germans or aliens or a very small sun.

THE MAN FROM HOLLOW EARTH

WHEN THE PEOPLE OF HOLLOW EARTH learned that the message of Admiral Byrd was withheld by the US Military they decided to send one of their own people to the surface world. Zaraya a native of Hollow Earth was one of the many actual eye witnesses to the presence of Admiral Byrd when he visited their world inside the Earth in the 1940s. And Zaraya was chosen to be the one to be sent to the surface world. But by sending people to the surface world requires some physical adjustments and transformation. And this includes shrinking the stature of Zaraya from 14 foot tall into the size of a human toddler. This may be difficult to understand from our own current knowledge of science. But the people of Hollow Earth they have advanced technology that goes back thousands and thousands of years ahead of ours here on the surface world. They put him on a chamber and then he started shrinking in size, transforming into a body of a child. In short, they modified his body in order to conform into how children looks like in our world.

In 1951, Zaraya who became a child was deposited in Texas and was adopted by the Woodard family. And that adoption gave him the name as Billie Faye Woodard.

The transformation have had some side effects though in the form of temporary slight amnesia. But as soon as Billie continue to grow and mature physically then his memory started to come back slowly. This was even more improved when his own father from Hollow Earth visited him while Billie was inside their kitchen. The name of his original father is Zorra. And Zorra appeared and helped his child remember the past and get him back in line to what his original mission for coming to the surface. Zorra used his own aeroship to come to the surface, but for us, we call it UFO.

One of the remarkable thing that makes Billie different from us here on the surface is that unlike us he does not have a blood type. His blood is different. It seems the composition of his blood is more advanced in the sense that any virus and or bacteria that was tested in the laboratory of the US Military could not infect his blood. Instead the virus and the bacteria died for some unknown reason when mixed with his own blood on a petri dish; and this was observed by doctors with their own microscope. Billie also does not have any fingerprints. All of his fingers does not have any skin threads that we associate as "human fingerprints". He does not have any of this, and this has been proven several times. And the another thing that makes him distinct from surface people is that he has a dual hearts. Instead of one; Billie has two hearts operating simultaneously in his chest as though one heart is not enough. But maybe there's a reason for that as it won't make you get tired too fast.

As of this moment Billie lives in the state of Nevada. Over the years there were plenty of people who interviewed him and none of them can find anything wrong with what he is saying as everything that he says are always consistent.

The following are some of the main message of Billie for the world:

Our Earth is Hollow. Advanced, benevolent civilizations live within our Earth and will soon be emerging and helping us through Earth's coming transition.

Nuclear fuels are exposing Earth's populations to harmful side effects and should be stopped.

Fossil fuels are also harmful contaminants and should be replaced with safe and natural energy.

All diseases are curable and can be avoided.

Many hearing these messages will soon be transitioning into 5th Dimension.

It is important for us to understand that we are Unlimited Beings and can reclaim our Godhood.

If you have noticed that there was an effective halt over the testing and use of nuclear weapons on the surface world for the last two to three decades. According to Billie the people of Hollow Earth along with the Galactics have been very active in stopping any nuclear armaments from being used. Even nuclear warheads that was secretly sent into space by NASA was stopped by them as they cannot allow the US Military to play with nuclear weapons. They have given them several warnings in the past but they just won't listen. The explosion in Nagasaki and Hiroshima was a warning sign for them to interfere to the affairs of the surface world, not in a violent or disrespectful way but for peace and for the good of everyone. Since, the surface world and the people of Hollow Earth share the same planet, every pollution including radiation that is emitted into the atmosphere of the world can also affect the atmosphere of those inside the Earth. As the north and south pole are actually open and anything in the wind can be carried into inside the Earth. And this is one of the many reason why they just cannot possibly allow any radiation to enter Hollow Earth's domain as those things can damage the natural ecological condition inside the Earth.

The people of Hollow Earth do have satellites operating in our atmosphere and they are there to observe what we are doing in this world. These satellites are situated in high and lower orbit. And with these satellites, they can then monitor the movements, communication of the secret government on the surface world and find out in real time what is going on in our world. In short, nothing escapes from the watchful eyes orbiting in space. They can scan the underground bunkers and see what the secret government is hiding underneath the Earth. But take note, this only acts like a CCTV camera and not there to control any of the lives of the people on the surface. In comparison to what the secret government of the world; they have more than 60 secret satellites in orbit some are facing the Earth and some are facing outward into the outer space. Guess who are they watching 24 hours a day that are coming and going from this planet? And yet we were conditioned to believe that we are alone in the universe. And they have been doing that for decades a decade without the knowledge of the people of the surface.

Right now Billie lives in the state of Nevada, if you have

questions go ahead and ask him. Either gives him a call or visit him in his home. He is here to help us understand and to awaken to the truth.

Going back to the story narrative. Billie eventually became a Colonel for the US Air Force. And he was stationed at Area 51. He was one of the people who tested to fly the back engineered UFOs that the military collected from several UFO crash sites in the United States and other parts of the world. And because of the secrecy, they are only allowed to fly those UFOs made by the US Air Force during night time. Yes, the story of Area 51 is true and that there was a coverup. In Area 51 there are several underground levels one of it leads to the Inner Earth or the crust of the Earth which is about 800 miles thickness. After the 800 miles solid crust is the Hollow interior space called "Hollow Earth". Inner Earth and Hollow Earth are not the same, but the people who lived in these two domains are the same in their principles of oneness as they live in unity and harmony.

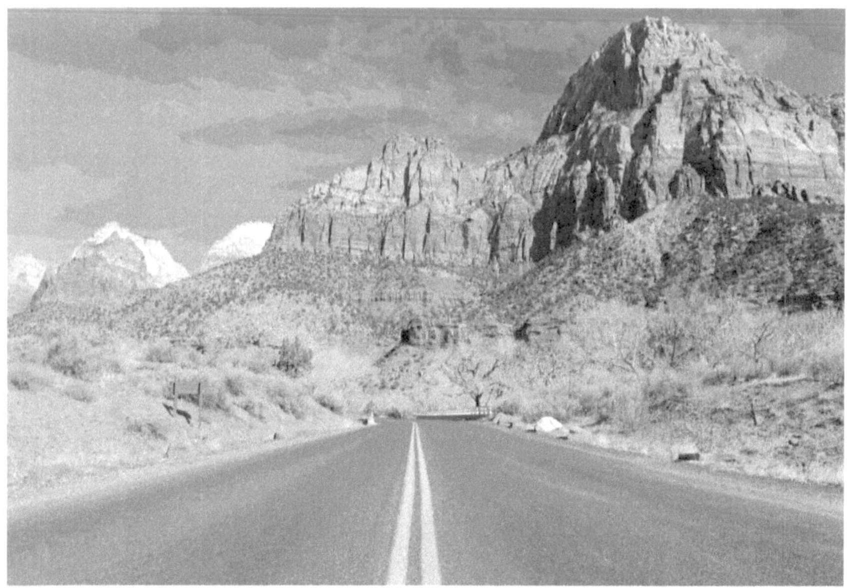

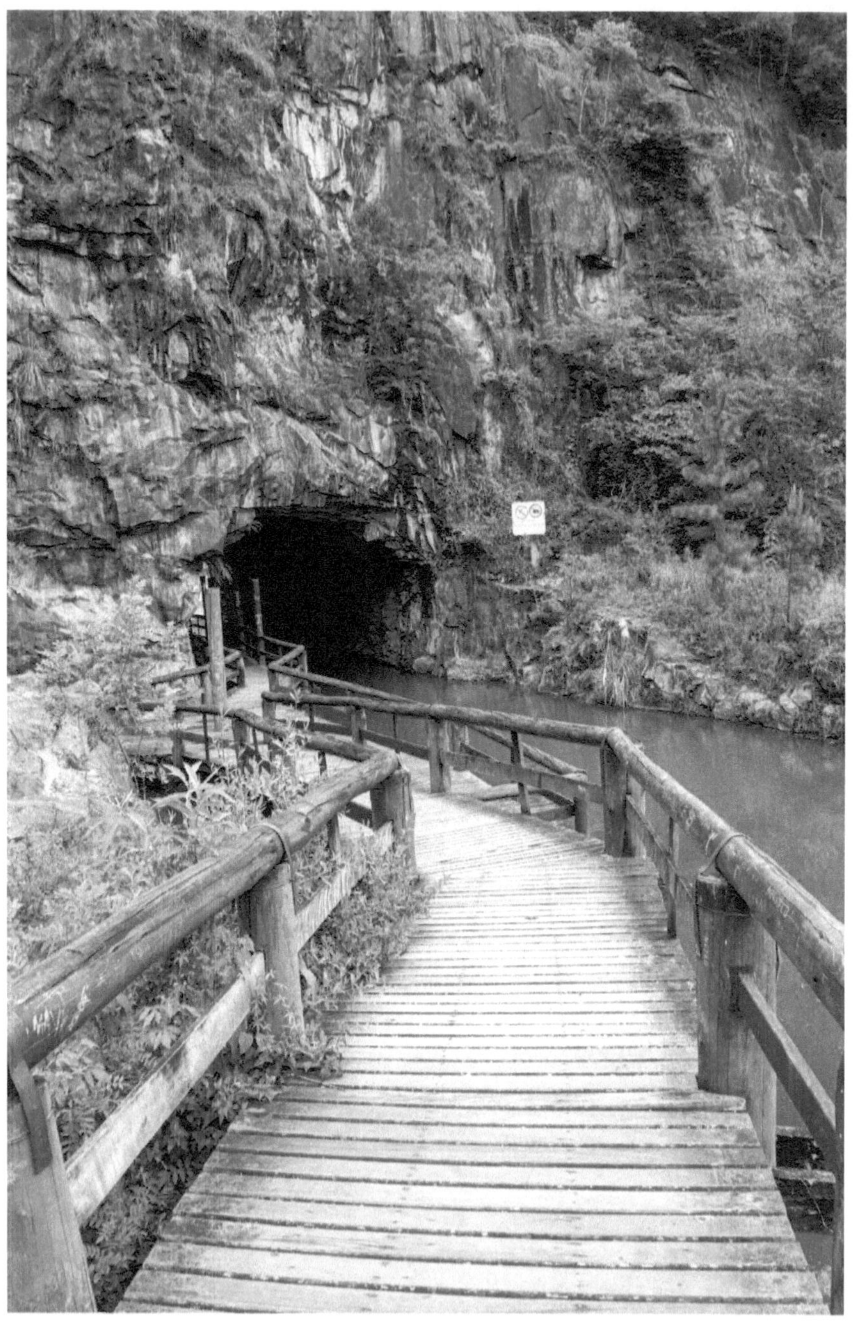

TRAVELER TO INNER EARTH

Arrival and Indoctrination

Upon my arrival to Area 51 I was indoctrinated to the existence of tunnels beneath Area 51, and soon after I met several of the Underground Shuttle Operators that have a stature of 13 to 14 feet in height. These tunnels, that transverse the world, are built by a species of beings who have existed here before we, a very long time.

Immediately on my arrival to Area 51, I was made aware of the tunnels and all the workings of the facility itself. They told me that the first 15 levels of the Area 51 facility were man made; that Levels 16-27 were already there. Nobody from our government made them. We were just facilitating them.

My father had been stationed at Roswell. As part of my induction into the military he requested that I be stationed along with him at the Pentagon. There they said "We have a new duty station for you which will be Area 51 facility, Nevada", Commonly referred to as S-4. When I went into the

Pentagon I was a Second Lieutenant.

When I came to the Pentagon they gave me the field commission as First Lieutenant. After 3 weeks of being there they handed me my full Colonel rank, saying "you have to be a full Colonel to be stationed at this next facility". There were 150,000 personnel in this facility, approx. 85% military personnel and 15% civilian. Following my arrival, I was taken underground and did not see the light of day for 11.5 years.

The Tunnels and Shuttles

The Walls of the Tunnels are very smooth. If you were to pull a hollow tube through a ball of clay you can get an idea of how smooth. The walls have what is likened to a marble finish, which are made of a metal substance, impenetrable; the surface of the walls cannot be penetrated even by a diamond drill nor will a laser penetrate the surface.

Remember there was a time when we used to see troop movements from point A to B on the Earth's surface, continually. It was not that long ago. Now, you rarely see this. Now they use tunnels to move all these troops at long distances. The tunnels are wide enough to drive two, 18 foot wheelers side by side.

Stemming from Area 51, one shuttle goes out to the Pacific Ocean - 350 miles due west of Monterey - where there is a pyramid; another shuttle goes to the Cheyenne Mountain facility

The length of a large shuttle machine is approx 1/4 mile long. Interior inhabitants make use of these machines - a huge vessel for moving large numbers of people/beings/whatever quickly.

The smaller shuttle is 50-60 feet in length, this was the kind I was in. The speed of the shuttles is faster than the speed of sound, they can travel from Area 51 to the main interior of the Earth in less than 10 Earth minutes. In 5-6 minutes you are there.

The material used to make the shuttles is the same substance that made up the skin of the spacecraft at Roswell. The shuttles run on electromagnetic power using the Earth's grid line. The operators who I mentioned earlier who are of a stature of 13-14 ft. in height, look like us in their appearance but much more highly evolved, and speak through telepathy. The men have beards or not, and the women's skin is flawless, indeed having a perfect clear complexion. Their expression for Humans is one of concern for Us - as they see where we Humans are headed. There are seven civilizations residing in the Inner Earth - which are governed by the principles of harmony. They understand and they speak all languages of the earth. Their understanding of medical knowledge is phenomenal.

Personal History

At the age of 12, while walking through a field of corn with another friend I had a paranormal experience. I was taken into a UFO vehicle and transported into the Inner Earth. Here, I lived for 6 months among the Hollow Earth residents.

You may imagine the wonder of my parents especially of my Father who was in the Military Service, at that time when I disappeared, then to mysteriously return in 6 months. It was due to this experience that I believe my Father made certain that I was engaged under his wing at the Pentagon and later directed to serve at Area 51.

I am not the biological offspring of my father, but an adopted child as was my sister. My sister and I were separated when she was put in the hands of the "secret government" for observation. They were trying to find the source of her paranormal abilities. When she became aware of their plans to take her life to perform a research autopsy, she sent a telepathic call to Hollow Earth and on her next "airing" on the surface, was swiftly picked up by one of the aero ships. I was able to combat their negativity with my mind, which is stronger, and survived their attacks.

My father, Zorra, is a Hollow Earth scientist who has made 150,000 trips around the sun. My sister and myself are originally from the Hollow Earth. Our true parents and family live in Hollow Earth. When our adoption father took us in as adopted children we spoke a language unknown to any surface culture.

I have an unknown blood type. I have never had a disease of any kind. My blood has been medically examined and destroys all viral infection when combined with other blood samples in a lab setting.

Hollow Earth Vortexes

The Hollow Earth residents have the ability to split the ocean floor and create a vortex, as is shown with the Bermuda Triangle. There are 7 different levels in these vortexes, and equipment and beings are brought in and placed corresponding to these different levels.

The vortexes act as doorways for entrance or exit to the hollow interior of the Earth. There is more than one triangle area off of Florida, one at Lake Erie, and another off the coast of Mexico, one off of Japan; as well as other geographic locations of the Earth. These are called "Quiet Zones". These doorways allow creatures from the interior to come out and in such as the Sasquatch, Lochness...etc.

All planets are Hollow as is the Sun, which is really a planet. There are civilizations in the Sun which have colonies in the Earth' subterranean regions.

Seeking Entry

In order to locate an entrance to the Inner Earth, where ever you are underground, all that you need is your compass. The compass will spin as if you are standing at the North Pole at the tunnel entrance to the Inner Earth.

When I left the Military Service, I no longer had a means of going into the Hollow Earth. It was necessary that I seek another way. I, and a party of interested seekers, rented a plane which took us to the very rim of the North Pole.

The People of the Interior

The people of the interior were very free with showing me around, very articulate in showing you what is exactly going on - they do not hold anything back. They always ask permission when working with Nature, they ask the plants for permission before consuming them or cutting them down, they ask the Mother Earth before they build on it, and do so build with the lay of the land which best suits their environment, a practice similar to the American Indians; therefore seeking to preserve a harmonious state at all times; wanting to be one with Nature at all times; they are more spiritually advanced than surface dwellers and greatly respect Mother Earth.

The atmosphere is crystal clear, as a rule there, are at times clouds, but nothing like rain clouds. The temperature is a constant 73 degrees.

The people in the interior speak directly with the animals and the animals speak directly to the people of the interior.

There is no need for hoarding, for everything is free, no need to create in abundance as everything is ample. A process of bartering is more common than trade in money.

This is basically a utopian culture with no depression leading into violence. No parties seeking to make war and gain dominance over each other. There are none richer nor poorer.

There are aero-ships (we term on the surface as flying saucers) in which a part of themselves, a part of their personality goes into the creation of the aero-ship through the process of thought, due to their very powerful minds. This makes the aero-ships perfect in design and execution in motion. Only a few persons of the surface have these similar abilities to create, due to the repression of these abilities in childhood by religion, education, and family fears. The people of the interior are allowed to enter the space of their imagination if you will, and there they create. Disease will not enter their bodies - for it is not allowed.

As surface Humanity enters into the coming 4th dimensional phase, the Inner Earth people will come forward and more deeply work with us on the surface. People on the surface are presently so involved with the sense of "me" that they cannot live together harmoniously.

People of the surface who seek to reach the Inner Earth

inhabitants through meditation will receive it. Children who are being born now are becoming more capable of using the wholeness of their brain, which is in common practice in the Interior.

One of the first things they showed us in the interior was their capability of interplanetary travel and time travel. The basis of time travel is likened to bending space, which comes through the power of meditation and by the acceptance of being an unlimited being. If you train your mind at a subconscious level that you are an unlimited being all things are possible.

On the surface, capabilities to experience this infinite power are more easily awakened at such Portals as Mt. Shasta which serves as a Space Time Portal directly to the Inner Earth. Once in the surroundings of Mt. Shasta you are drawn into the "harmonious state". In my experiences at Mt. Shasta, the Telosians in their civilisation underground in that area are projecting an aura of great harmony in a lovely atmosphere.

Area 51

Of all I saw at Area 51, 95% remains hidden from the public. Going into Area 51 is like going into another world, where they are terribly afraid that other countries and other parties are going to get "this" information. Their thoughts being "if we admit that the Earth is Hollow, with a central intelligence in it, this is going to cause discord and fear". This fear process is generated by the private companies who seek to control and advance their own needs and personal agendas through Area 51.

I left the Air Force due to their domineering ways by those who sought to act like control freaks, who were stagnating my ability to think and act in a creative manner. In accepting their Orders not to talk about such information, they take it for granted that one will automatically obey.

Because of my outgoing desire to share information and inform the public at large my Service Pension and all my benefits and rights such as the use of the Commissary, dental and medical, were taken away.

I was in the military for 13.5 years, from basic to the Pentagon and then to Area 51. The genetic engineering that is taking place at Area 51 is with our younger generation. The "milk carton children" whose photos were commonly seen in the markets in the past, were abducted and taken to Area 51.

Level 16 of Area 51 is the genetic engineering level, where they are using our children for experimentation in longevity and powers of the mind. The major force behind this is what is termed as the "Secret Government". There are civilians of the Secret Government which are in control in several areas of Area 51.

There is a network of tunnels underground that go all the way to Europe, South America - the several continents. And there is an intermingling of this great network of tunnels throughout the globe, of which many governments use. God bless you and be with you.

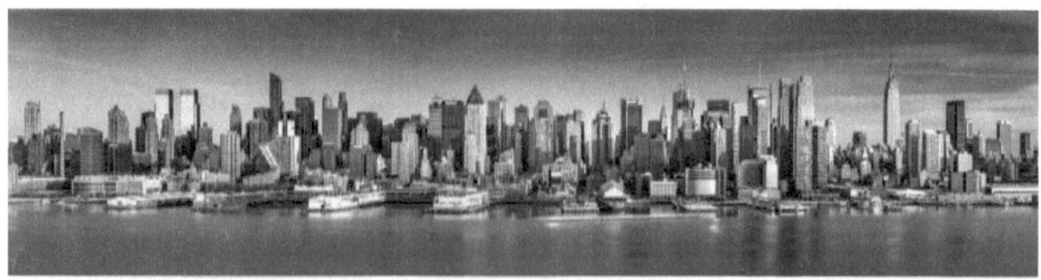

BENEFITS OF THE AGE PILL

HOW IT WORK

The Age Pill works in 3 extremely powerful ways by removing glycogen buildups that inhibit intercellular proteins from performing their DNA repair functions.

Secondly, the Age Pill supports the stem cell's internal system to break down and remove toxins, sludge and cellular garbage that has built up, allowing the body to repair itself. Also, by cleaning the pathways of the brain, it allows the neural transmitters to function more efficiently.

Lastly, the Age Pill allows a significant increase in ATP, prefacing biological hydrogen.

The hydrogen atom becomes the "glue" mechanism for your DNA resulting in the repairing of cells that increases electrical energy within the stem cells by as much as four times, providing a noticeable increase in energy levels and body metabolism resulting in excess weight loss and overall alertness.

- Improved Sleep

- Nail Growth

- Improved Mood

- More Motivation

- Improved Energy

- Improved Mental Clarity

- Improved Libido

- Varicose And Spider Veins

- Improved Stamina

- Weight Loss

- Changes In Vision

- Hair Color Returning

- Changes In Aging Skin

- Less Hair Loss

- Improved Metabolism

- Thicker/Fuller Hair

- Auto-Immune Support

- Chronic Fatigue Support

• Depression Support

• Lyme Damage Repair

•Adrenal Health Support

• Improved Gastrointestinal Issues.

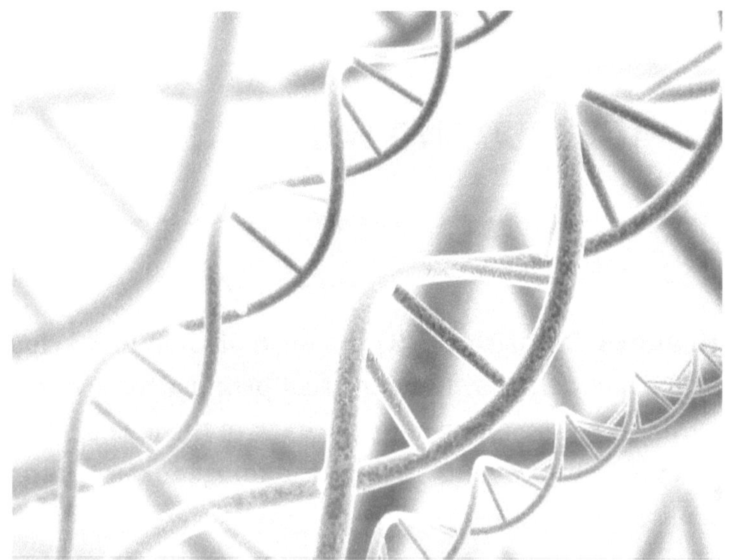

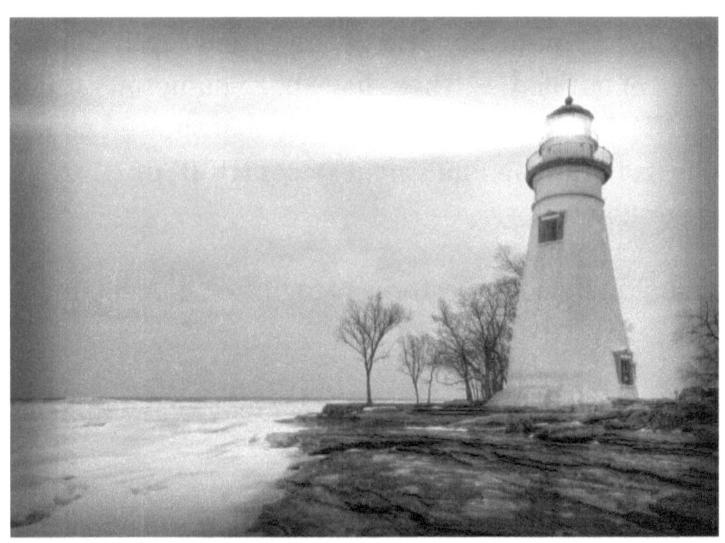

AGE PILL AND WHAT THEY DO

Nicotinamide Riboside- (NR) is a form of vitamin B3 closely related to Niacin that is showing great promise for it's ability to raise NAD+ levels in older humans, back to the levels normally found in youth to prevent and repair damage to various organs in the body.

NAD+ (Nicotinamide Adenine Dinucleotide) is a key co-enzyme that enables the mitochondria to power and repair damage in every cell of our bodies. There have been numerous studies of NR and NMN supplementation in mice that showed no negative side effects in Human Equivalent Doses (HED) of 2.1 to 17 grams per day.

Nicotinamide Riboside restores recognition in Alzheimers Mice.

Nicotinamide Riboside improves metabolic health in mice exposed to a high fat diet.

NAD+ repletion improves stem cell function and enhances life span in mice.

Research shows Nicotinamide Riboside prevents liver cancer in mice.

Nicotinamide Riboside reverses Fatty Liver Disease in Mice.

Nicotinamide Riboside Opposes Type 2 Diabetes and Neuropathy in Mice.

The FDA recently granted Nicotinamide Riboside GRAS (Generally Recognized as Safe) status on the basis of this clinical study, which showed "no observed adverse effect level was 300 mg/kg/day."

Beta-Alanine- is a naturally occurring beta amino acid that is converted to other chemicals that can then affect the muscles. This has been shown to enhance muscular endurance. Beta-Alanine supplementation can also improve moderate to high intensity cardiovascular exercise performance, like rowing or sprinting. When beta-alanine is ingested, it turns into the molecule carnosine, which acts as an acid buffer in the body. Carnosine is stored in cells and releases in response to drops in the pH. Increased stores of carnosine can protect against diet induced drops in the pH as well as offer protection from exercise induced lactic acid production. Carnosine also shows reduction of oxidative stress and glycation products. Rated one of the number one protein supplements for muscle support.

Alpha-Lipoic acid-(ALA) -is found in the body and also synthesized by plants and animals. Its present in every cell of the body and helps turn glucose into fuel for the body to run off of. Its most valuable role is fighting the effects of free radicals which are dangerous chemical reaction byproducts that form during the process of oxidation. Within our cells, ALA is converted into dihydrolipoic acid, which has protective effects over normal cellular reactions. Like other antioxidants ALA can help to slow down cellular damage that is one of the root causes of diseases like cancer, heart disease and diabetes. It also works in the body to restore essential vitamin levels, such as Vit E and Vit C, along with helping the body digest and utilize carbohydrate molecules while turning them into usable energy. ALA is both water soluble and fat soluble unlike other nutrients which can only be properly absorbed with either one or the other. There is some evidence that ALA acts as a heavy metal chelator, binding metals in the body. ALA can increase how the body uses glutathione, and it might increase energy metabolism as well- which is why this supplement is often used by athletes to enhance physical performance. ALA can protect cells and neurons involved in hormone production, one benefit is it offers protection against diabetes. Because alpha lipoic acid can protect cells and neurons involved in hormone production, one benefit is it offers protection against diabetes. ALA is considered an effective drug in the treatment of diabetic distal sensory- motor neuropathy, which affects about 50 percent of people with diabetes. (5) In dietary supplement form, ALA seems to help improve insulin sensitivity and might also offer protection against metabolic syndrome a term given to a cluster of conditions like high blood pressure, cholesterol and body weight. Some evidence also shows that it can help lower blood sugar levels. ALA is used to help relieve complications and symptoms of diabetes caused by nerve damage, including numbness in the legs and arms, cardiovascular problems, eye-related disorders, pain, and swelling. That's why it should be part of any diabetic diet plan to treat this common disorder.

People who experience peripheral neuropathy as a side effect of diabetes can find relief from pain, burning, itching, tingling and numbness using ALA, although most studies show that high doses in IV form are most effective as opposed to eating ALA-rich foods. A major benefit of alpha lipoic supplementation in diabetics is the lowered risk for neuropathic complications that affect the heart, since around 25 percent of people with diabetes develop cardiovascular autonomic neuropathy (CAN). CAN is characterized by reduced heart rate variability and is associated with an increased risk of mortality in people with diabetes. Oxidative stress can damage nerves in the eyes and cause vision problems, especially in people with diabetes or older adults. Alpha lipoic acid has been used successfully to help control symptoms of eye-related disorders, including vision loss, macular degeneration, retina damage, cataracts, glaucoma and Wilson's disease. Results from certain studies demonstrate that long-term use of alpha lipoic acid has beneficial effects on the development of retinopathy since it halts oxidative damage that can result in modified DNA in the retina.

DMAE- (dimethylaminoethanol) is a substance naturally produced in small amounts in the brain and also found in anchovies and sardines. DMAE supplements are promoted to boost brainpower, improve memory, and slow aging. The idea that DMAE can improve memory stems from research suggesting it may increase levels of the neurotransmitter acetylcholine, which is believed to play an important role in learning and memory. Levels of acetylcholine decline among people with Alzheimer's disease, and the drugs used to treat Alzheimer's patients target the processes that break it down. DMAE has also been studied as a means of relieving the symptoms of tardive dyskinesia, a spastic disorder that is a side-effect of long-term use of some anti-psychotic medications. Despite some promising preliminary studies, subsequent research failed to confirm that DMAE had any effect. DMAE Bitartrate is a powdered form of the compound Dimethylaminoethanol (also known as DMAE or Deanol), a naturally occurring compound in the brain. DMAE is a precursor to the neurotransmitter choline. Choline has been shown to directly influence the areas of learning and memory.

 DMAE bitartrate is particularly beneficial for your memory function cal also increase mental adaptability, concentration, brain cell health and give you better analytic processing skills as well. DMAE is a compound that is known as a mind health compound. It does this by reducing buildup of what is known as the 'age pigment', which impairs cognitive function and is implicated in the cognitive decline with age. It can also increase levels of the compound involved with memory, acetylcholine. It can also protect neurons and other cells from harmful effects of certain types of oxidation by embedding itself in the structure of the cell and acting as an antioxidant, as well as sustaining metabolic processes in the body through a process known as 'methyl donation'. DMAE is also found in various face and body creams, and can tighten and tone skin quality.

L-Carnosine (beta-alanyl-L-histidine), featuring the characteristic Imidazole- ring, is a dipeptide molecule, made up of the amino acids beta-alanine and histidine. It is highly concentrated in muscle and brain tissues. Carnosine acts as an anti-glycating agent, reducing the rate of formation of advanced glycation end- products (AGEs) (substances that can be a factor in the development or worsen of many degenerative diseases, such as diabetes, atherosclerosis, chronic renal failure, and Alzheimer's disease), and ultimately reducing development of atherosclerotic plaque build-up. Chronic glycolysis is speculated to accelerate aging, making carnosine a candidate for therapeutic potential. L-carnosine, sometimes called simply carnosine, is a combination of two amino acids, alanine and histidine. Your body manufactures carnosine, found in high concentrations in skeletal muscle, the lenses of the eyes, the brain and the nervous system. Carnosine acts as an antioxidant, a substance that neutralizes free radicals, which damage cells. potential benefits on the fact that carnosine inhibits advanced glycation end products, called AGEs, which contribute to Alzheimer's disease. One study found that in rat lenses exposed to substances that induce cataract formation and carnosine, carnosine prevented or reversed cataracts (Biochemistry study 5/14/2009). L-Carnosine may be recommended as an adjunct therapy for diabetes mellitus or autism. This supplement has also been researched for its antiglycation, antioxidant, cardioprotective, anticancer and antidiabetic effects. In humans, carnosine is naturally found in the brain, skeletal muscles, the heart and certain other innervated organs and tissues. Supports athletic performance and muscle vitality as well. A number of experiments carried out in Australia showed that Carnosine reinvigorates cells as they approach senescence (the stage just before they die when the cell is not functioning). Cells were given Carnosine actually looked and behaved younger than untreated cell's. Importantly, Carnosine reversed the signs of aging in these senescent (nearly dead) cells.

This means that Carnosine is a great for older people who want to look younger, as well as those who want to continue looking younger. Carnosine limits the formation of oxidized sugars, commonly known as Advanced Glycosylation End-products (AGEs) by acting as an antioxidant. From an anti-aging perspective, the fewer AGEs created in your body the better. Carnosine prevents lipid, DNA, and protein damage by removing harmful metals via chelation. Carnosine may prevent Alzheimer's by counteracting the buildup of aldehydes and amyloid plaques, which are widely considered to be the primary causes of Alzheimer's. The aggregation of beta amyloid into fibrillar structures contributed to Alzheimer's disease. Carnosine was found to impede the formation of fibrillar structures by altering the hydrogen bond network involved in fibrillogenesis. By protecting the brain against free radicals and advanced glycation end products carnosine may provide a useful tool for tackling Alzheimer's.

Betaine Hcl-Betaine hydrochloride is an acidic form of betaine, a vitamin-like substance found in grains and other foods. Betaine hydrochloride is recommended by some doctors as a supplemental source of hydrochloric acid for people who have a deficiency of stomach acid production (hypochlorhydria). In biological systems, many naturally occurring betaines serve as organic osmolytes, substances synthesized or taken up from the environment by cells for protection against osmotic stress, drought, high salinity or high temperature. Intracellular accumulation of betaines, non-perturbing to enzyme function, protein structure, and membrane integrity, permits water retention in cells, thus protecting from the effects of dehydration. It is also a methyl donor of increasingly recognized significance in biology.

Acetyl L-carnitine. Acetyl L-carnitine (ALC) is an amino acid that's primarily used by the body for energy production but also helps create acetylcholine, a brain chemical associated with memory and cognitive function. * It's been shown to help mental fatigue associated with aging.* Acetyl-L-Carnitine is an amino acid the body uses to turn fat into energy. It is not normally considered an essential nutrient because the body can manufacture all it needs. However, supplemental Carnitine may improve the ability of certain tissues to produce energy. This effect has led to the use of Carnitine in various muscle diseases as well as heart conditions. Additionally, a preliminary study suggests that Carnitine may be useful for improving blood sugar control in individuals with type 2 (adult-onset) diabetes. It also might help prevent diabetic cardiac autonomic neuropathy (injury to the nerves of the heart caused by diabetes). Weak evidence suggests that Carnitine may be able to improve cholesterol and triglyceride levels, and also help individuals with degeneration of the cerebellum (the structure of the brain responsible for voluntary muscular movement). One very small study suggests Carnitine may be helpful for reducing symptoms of chronic fatigue syndrome.

One study suggests that Carnitine may be of value for treating hyperthyroidism. Acetyl L-carnitine Hcl is a potent super nutrient that supports the body in the same wat as L-carnitine but also has the ability to pass through the blood brain barrier. Supports mental sharpness by stimulating acetylcholine production. It has been shown to help maintain cellular stability and to promote cell membrane health. Acetyl L-Carnitine HCL Research Cellular energy production itself produces free radicals that can harm cell structures, including the mitochondria, if the body's natural antioxidant capacity is low. Acetyl l- carnitine and lipoic acid are both naturally present antioxidants in the body that have been shown to support mitochondrial function and help reduce free radical damage. (Hagen TM et al., 1998; Lyckesfeldt J et al., 1998) Acetyl l-carnitine HCL enhances energy production by promoting the transport of fatty acids into the energy-producing units in the cells. In two animal studies from the University of California at Berkeley (Hagen TM et al., 1998) acetyl l-carnitine significantly benefited mitochondrial health and promoted increased cellular respiration and membrane health.

L-5-Hydroxytryptophan-5-HTP is the precursor of the neurotransmitter serotonin. 5- HTP is obtained from the seeds of the plant Griffonia simplicifolia. also known as oxitriptan (INN), is a naturally occurring amino acid and chemical precursor as well as a metabolic intermediate in the biosynthesis of the neurotransmitter serotonin. 5-HTP has been suggested as a treatment for many conditions. Some research supports the use of 5-HTP in treating cerebellar ataxia, headache, depression, psychiatric disorders, and fibromyalgia, and as an appetite suppressant or weight loss agent. Parkinson's disease is a neurological disorder that usually develops around the age of 50. The disorder occurs when the brain cells that make dopamine slowly degenerate. Symptoms includes tremors (shaking) and difficulties with movement and coordination. 5-HTP has been studied, usually in combination with drugs, for Parkinson's disease. Widely used to help with obesity (dieting), PMS, migraines, depression, anxiety, insomnia and addictive behavior. 5 HTP increases production of serotonin. Serotonin levels in the nervous system are essential for so many aspects of our daily lives. Serotonin is responsible for feelings of wellbeing, satisfaction and for normal sleep patterns. Obesity, PMS, migraines, depression, anxiety, insomnia and addictive behavior have all been associated with low levels of serotonin. Serotonin plays an important role in controlling anger, aggression, body temperature, mood, sleep, human sexuality, appetite, and metabolism, as well as stimulating vomiting. Clinical studies have shown that supplementing with 5-HTP produces positive results in weight loss, anxiety and depression.

Blueberry Fruit-They protect our bodies from damage by free radicals, unstable molecules that can damage cellular structures and contribute to aging and diseases like cancer. Blueberries are believed to contain the highest antioxidant capacity of ALL commonly consumed fruits and vegetables. The main antioxidant compounds in blueberries belong to a large family of polyphenols, called flavonoids. One group of flavonoids in particular, anthocyanins, is thought to be responsible for much of the beneficial health effects. They have been shown to directly increase antioxidant levels inside the body. Because blueberries are high in antioxidants, they can help neutralize some of the free radicals that cause damage to our DNA.

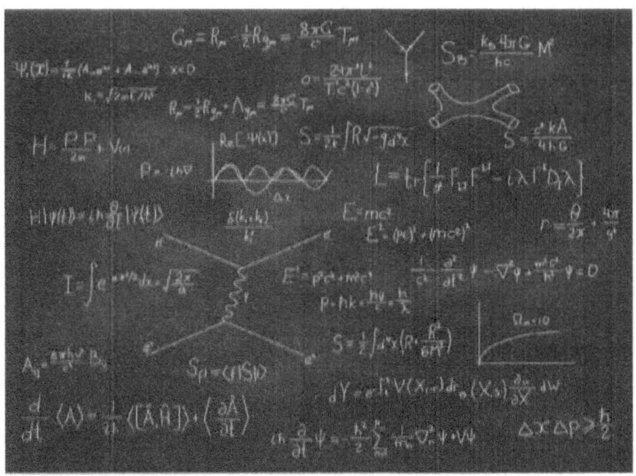

THE SCIENCE BEHIND THE AGE PILL

Age Reversal

The AGE Pill is about the closest thing to the fountain of youth that modern science has been able to produce so far. If you're into anti-ageing and would like to have your metabolic markers return to where they were in your 20's then what you're about to read is for you.

Glycation and Ageing

The term AGE is actually an acronym for "Anti Glycation Extreme". So what is glycation? Glycation is what occurs when blood glucose molecules bond with protein molecules in our bodies. The pathological impact of that unavoidable phenomenon is the formation of something called an advanced glycation end product. This happens to all of us … slowly … over a lifetime.

As children we had all the energy we needed, all day long. This energy is derived from metabolizing glucose sugar. As our bodies break down the glucose, the oxidation process releases the energy that powers the cells in our body. But unfortunately, a plaque-like residue is left over and forms a coating over the cells. This oxidized glucose plague is called "glycation".

You can observe the effects of acute glycation in diabetes patients. People suffering from diabetes tend to age faster and along with that, they experience the early onset of degenerative diseases. This is due to poor sugar control.

At some level, the same thing is happening to every single one of us – just not to the same extreme, nor at the same rate. So in short, "glycation" is the result of lifelong glucose exposure – the metabolism of which is essential for life and energy, but it comes with this pathological "side effect". The buildup of this plaque-like substance also interferes with inter-cellular (cell-to-cell) communication.

The Vital Role of Stem Cells

Now let's talk briefly about stem cells. When we are young, our bodies grow quickly. We have an abundance of stem cells which are highly productive. These stem cells are the "master cells" in our bodies that are able to transform into any type of cell that we need. As we grow, the stem cells divide and multiply into the trillions of cells that comprise an adult body. Our stem cells also replace the cells in our bodies that wear out.

But when glycation occurs and plaque-like metabolized glucose residues attach themselves to the proteins in our stem cells, they create a kind of "barrier" or film over the stem cells, so that they slowly lose their efficiency and functionality. As a consequence, a cellular "sludge" forms inside the cells over time. The scientific name for this is "lipofuscin".

This lipofuscin 'sludge' buildup interferes with intra-cellular communication, both in our 'regular' cells, as well as our stem cells, so that they can no longer do the job they are supposed to do. As a consequence, the cell mitochondria are damaged – and because the mitochondria are like the "nuclear power plants" of our cells, we then find ourselves lacking energy.

Lack of energy and slowing down of regular bodily functions are the typical symptoms of ageing lack of muscle strength, memory loss etc. Cell regeneration is inhibited, so that we no longer create as many cells as we lose in a day. This is what ageing is. Ageing is not a disease it is a process.

To reverse ageing, we need a way to get back to 1:1 cell regeneration and efficient cell functionality. This is how it used to be when you were 20-25. Once you cross the 30 year old threshold, you begin to lose more cells than you create and the cells that you do have don't function internally as efficiently as they used to.

When lipofuscin caused by glycation is removed; when the cellular garbage is taken out of the stem cells, the mitochondria within the cells now have the ability to react by creating massive amounts of energy molecules and ATP-providing biological hydrogen which combines with the electrical energy of the body to make you feel like you have the energy of a teenager once again.

It doesn't happen overnight. It's a process but most people are experiencing noticeable result within a month, especially if they drink plenty of water (which aids in the flushing out process).

Adenosine Triphosphate (ATP) and biological hydrogen are believed to be the keys in supporting the releases of vast stores of energy that are available to your body. Your new, elevated energy can help your cells to rebuild, rejuvenate and provide an environment to work at more optimum levels. Potentially providing support to alleviate the ravages to our bodies that occur over our lifetime.

Science Discovers the Significant Role of NAD+

Researchers at Harvard Medical School and the University of New South Wales discovered a natural compound that reverses the cumulative effects of aging ….. NAD+

In a paper published in Science Today, the team identifies a critical step in the molecular process that allows cells to repair damaged DNA.

Their experiments in mice suggest that a treatment is possible for DNA damage from ageing and radiation. It is so promising it has attracted the attention of NASA, which believes this new discovery can help its mission to Mars program.

While our cells have the innate capability to repair DNA damage which happens every time we go out into the sun, for example their ability to do this declines as we age.

The scientists identified that the metabolite NAD+, which is naturally present in every cell of our body, plays a key role as a regulator in protein-to-protein interactions that control DNA repair.

Treating mice with a NAD+ precursor, or "booster" called NMN was shown to improved their cells' ability to repair DNA damage caused by radiation exposure or old age.

The A.G.E. Pill is the first to bring a complete NAD+ boosting nutraceutical product to market containing these exciting new anti-aging discoveries:- NAD+ precursor NR and proprietary supporting ingredients which the body readily converts into NAD+.

The pharmaceutical version of an NAD+ booster is at least 3-

5 years away and will likely be significantly more expensive after Human Trials, FDA approvals, and the legal patent process. Many of the scientists involved in the Harvard and UNSW research are already taking NAD+ boosting nutritional supplements just like those contained in Sisel's A.G.E. Pill.

How The Age Pill Reverses Ageing

According to The AGE Pill scientist and formulator, Tom Mower, it provides four classes of advanced super-nutrients, which provide intense support for:

Removing glycation plaque buildup that inhibit inter-cellular proteins.

Supporting the stem cells' internal system in breaking down the toxins and the cellular garbage that has built up and stimulating the creation of new stem cells.

Cleaning up and reactivating 'senile' stem cells, allowing them to produce ATP-providing biological hydrogen, for energy. Theoretically, this could increase the electrical energy within our stem cells by 3-4 times, to a point where you might feel like you were 20 again

Improves DNA repair processes via stimulating the production of NAD+

This can lead to toto spectacular results in weight loss, vision, hearing, blood pressure, organ repair, arthritis, diabetes, and many other issues. Within about 10 days to 2 weeks a person's stem cells can be overhauled and repaired at the DNA molecular level.

Directions For Use Of The AGE Pill

Take 6 capsules daily on an empty stomach 3 capsules in the morning and 3 capsules in the evening, or 2 capsules, 3 times daily. For faster results, it is recommended to "double-dose" for the first month, then back off to the regular "6 capsules per day" maintenance dose.

Some have experienced what is called a "niacin rush" when double-dosing. It's like that flushed feeling you get when you're embarrassed and you can feel your ears burning. It's completely harmless though. Drink plenty of water if this happens to you. In fact, for best results, drink plenty of water anyway.

Want to really push back against the effects of time? The AGE Pill 2 pack gives you more of this powerful product for less. Use it to extend your regimen or to share your secret with family or friends. After all, feeling great is best when shared with others!

Warning: Do not take if pregnant, nursing, or under 18 years old. If you are taking prescription medication, or have a pre-existing medical condition, consult your healthcare provider before taking this product. Keep out of the reach of children. Do not use if tamper evident ring or seal is broken. This product may cause temporary reddening of the skin or flushing.

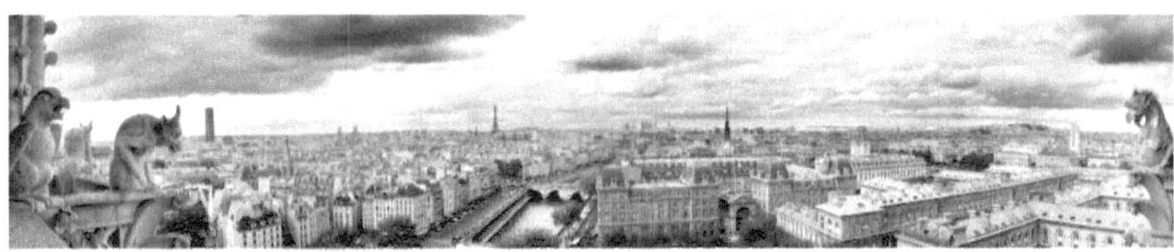

THE AGE PILL'S SUPERNUTRIENTS ACCELERATE

WHEN WE WERE VERY YOUNG, our bodies grew quickly, with an abundance of highly active stem cells. Stem cells are the master cells in our bodies that are able to transform into any type of cell that we need. As we grew, our stem cells divided and multiplied into the trillions of cells that make up an adult body, and replaced the cells in our body faster than they wore out and were discarded.

As children, we also had all of the energy that we needed to go all day long. This energy is derived from metabolizing glucose sugars to create electrical energy. As our bodies break glucose down through oxidation to release the energy that powers the cells in our body, a plaque like residue was left over. This residue known as AGE (Advanced Glycation End-products) accumulates over time, depositing an inhibiting coating over proteins, reducing optimal stem cell performance.

As the stem cells rebuild new cells and maintain themselves, Lipofuscin is formed. Lifofuscin is metabolic waste, a cellular sludge that builds up over our lifetime that clutters cells and greatly inhibits biological functions. It is difficult for our cells to produce the energy they need when this thick sludge inhibits flow and function.

But what if we got some help to clean up the mess and dump much of the accumulated trash left behind by glycation and lipofuscin? Then the stem cells in our bodies should be free to function again at a high level. Scientists now theorize it may well allow our bodies to again produce energy at the same levels as when we were in our prime, much like if we were in our 20's again.

This is what sets the AGE Pill™ apart from other anti-aging products, into the realm of potential youthful regeneration. The AGE Pill™ provides three classes of advanced, specialized super-nutrients to the stem cells to delivering intense support for:

Removing glycation plaque build-up that inhibit intercellular proteins.

Reduction/removal of toxins and cellular sludge resulting from biological activity creating lipofuscin.

Significantly increasing ATP-providing Biological Hydrogen to greatly amplify cellular electrical energy. Theoretically, this process could increase electrical energy within the stem cells three or fourfold, to where you may "feel like you were 20 again!"

Adenosine Triphosphate (ATP) and biological hydrogen are believed to be key in supporting the releases of vast stores of electrical energy to your body. Your enhanced, elevated energy could help your cells to rebuild, rejuvenate and work at more optimum levels, potentially alleviating the ravages to our bodies that occur over our lifetime.

Our powerful and unique synergistic blend, potentially maximizes The A.G.E. Pill's nutritional content, providing intense support for removing glycation buildup, reducing toxins and increasing ATP, helping you look and feel like you were in your 20's again.

Supplements That Prevent Aging

When explorers first arrived in the new world, rumors abounded of a mythical fountain whose water was said to give one eternal youth. Though many hopeful searchers spent their lives in pursuit of this fantasy, in the end, they became old and past quietly into history. Today, rumors have returned about a "fountain of youth", but this time they aren't based on myth, but come from solid scientific research.

As science digs deeper and deeper into genetic research, more and more evidence emerges that humans do not have to age as they do. Research suggests that humans can essentially live forever given the proper conditions. Though science has many years ahead of it before it can truly stop the aging process, several nutritional supplements that prevent aging have been discovered. New discoveries arrive almost daily lending credibility to the effectiveness of certain supplements in slowing the aging process and anyone interested in staying young and healthy should investigate the findings. Here are a few of the best supplements available today to combat aging.

CoQ10 (Coenzyme Q10)

This is an enzyme that has numerous beneficial effects on the body. It is a powerful antioxidant that is especially effective in preventing heart disease. CoQ10 acts on every cell in the body and aid in energy production and cell rejuvenation. Evidence suggests that this enzyme is also very effective against breast cancer.

Resveratrol

Resveratrol is the chemical upon which scientists are staking their hopes for a true anti-aging drug. This is the age preventing chemical found in red wine, which has gotten so much press over the years as an antioxidant, heart saver and cance fighter. Resveratrol is available in pill and contrary to popular belief, you would have to drink much more red wine than your body could tolerate in order to derive the anti-aging and health benefits of Resveratrol, anyway.

Vitamin E

This is perhaps one of the first supplements giving credit for preventing aging. It consists of a number of powerful antioxidant compounds that aid in cell repair and have been proven to prevent and fight cancer. Though supplementation of vitamin E is recommended, care must be taken since high levels of vitamin E can be toxic.

Vitamin C

Most people have heard of vitamin C in its role in the prevention of the common cold. though that has recently been disputed, its role as an all around age preventing supplement is gaining momentum. It is another antioxidant that plays a role in cellular repair throughout the body. Vitamin C is water soluble and therefore is virtually impossible to take too much. Though available in supplement form, it is best when found in fresh fruits and vegetables.

Ease of Taking Supplements

Supplements by design are one of the easiest things that you can do to slow down the aging process. And many of these supplements not only help reverse the aesthetic effects of aging, but also the biological effects that aging has on organ systems and overall health.

This small list is just a drop in the ocean of age preventing supplements available today. Some of these supplements have scientifically proven track records while others are still being investigated.

Safety of Supplements

Consumers should research supplements before taking them to ensure they are right for their particular situation. If in doubt, individuals should check with their doctors prior to beginning a supplement regimen. Some supplements can interfere with medications that you may be taking, minimizing their effects or rendering them useless. It is especially important to check with your doctor before taking any type of supplement if you have a major health issue.

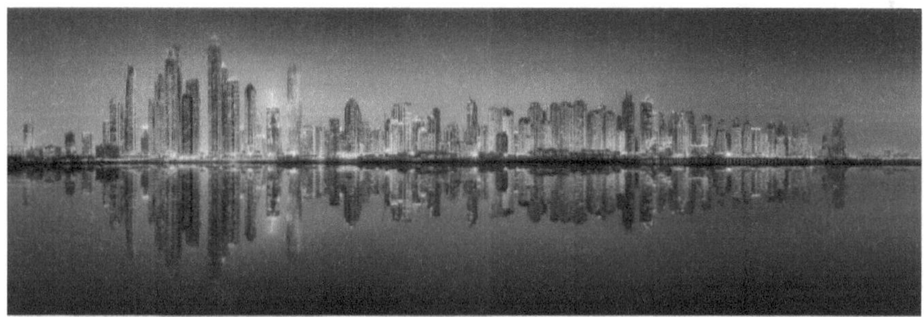

NUTRIENTS FOR HEALTHY SKIN

Do You Know What Your Body Is Missing?

It seems every time you turn your head, you see a new skin care cream. However, do you know that not all such products are good? Only the products consist of nutrients for healthy skin are effective for the skin. Well, what are these nutrients for healthy skin? How do they work and how can one achieve them?

Here is an article, which not only introduces you to the nutrients for healthy skin but also brings you up to speed with their sources.

Amino Acids & Peptides

Experts say that these two nutrients are an absolute must for the skin because they are the raw material for skin cells to produce collagen and elastin. We all know that collagen and elastin are required to make skin wrinkle free and smooth.

Minerals & Vitamins

Vitamins like C, D, K, E and minerals like Keratin are necessary for the wellbeing of skin cells. Skin cells remain healthier and live longer in their presence. Therefore, it is a must for an effective skin care cream to have these nutrients for healthy skin.

The immediate question you might have it that what are their sources? And how can one acquire them for a healthy skin? Read on to find out.

Food and Drinks

Vegetables like Spinach, Broccoli, Tomatoes, and Berries are rich source of minerals. Fruits like Banana, Oranges, Grape Fruit and Apple are rich source of vitamins. Green tea is a very good antioxidant, and helps maintain the health of skin cells. You can procure all these foods easily and can change your lifestyle to include them in your diet.

Skin Care Products

Natural products, which are made using natural ingredients are a good source of nutrients for healthy skin. Such products consist of ingredients like CynergyTK, Phytessence Wakame, CoenzymeQ10, Nano-Lipobelle H-EQ10, Avocado Oil, and many other natural emollients. These products are safe because these ingredients are derived from natural source, hence do not pose any danger to skin or any other body part.

In a nutshell, without these nutrients, your skin will not be as healthy as you want it to be. You might use products and consume pills but without these essential ingredients, you will never be able to attain a smooth and soft skin. For best results, learn more about natural products by reading about them on the internet. Once you are satisfied with the ingredients, then only make the buying decision.

Trust me, natural products are the only viable means of reversing the clock on aging skin and keeping it young forever.

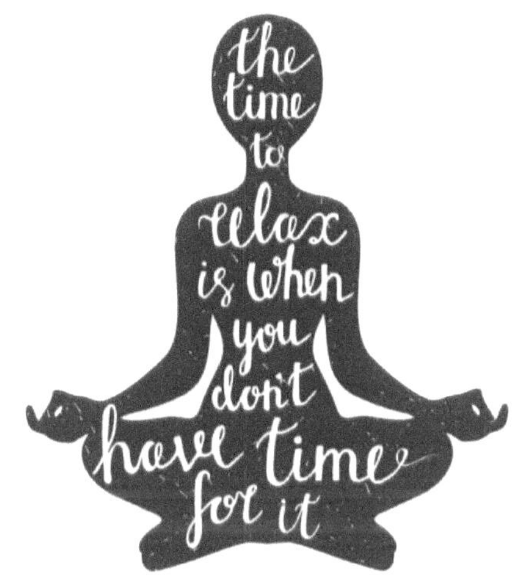

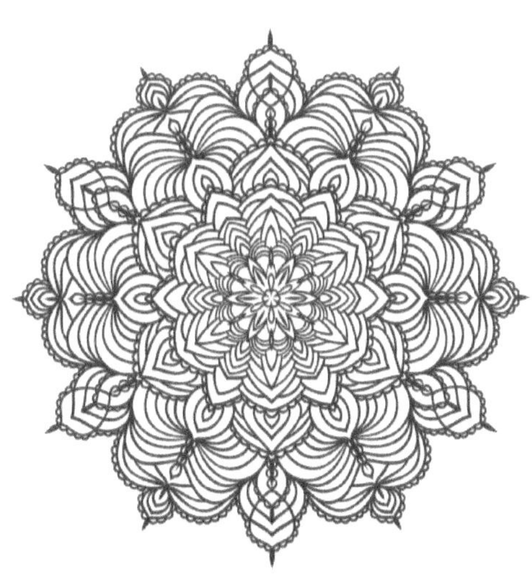

NATURAL HORMONE BALANCE

HORMONE BALANCE IS ESSENTIAL to healthy living. There is so much to understand about balancing hormones that it is difficult to know where to begin. Hormones are messengers in the body that travels through the bloodstream into the organs, lymph, and tissues of our bodies. The endocrine glands secrete certain hormones in the body which includes the pineal gland, pituitary, pancreas, thyroid, ovaries or testes, parathyroid, hypothalamus, adrenals and gastrointestinal tract. Just small hormonal changes can cause significant physiological changes in the body, including weight gain and forgetfulness.

Smart health is to have your hormone levels tested periodically, just like a mammogram or Pap smear. Imbalances have serious consequences and if not kept in check, chances of cancer increase, as well as other diseases like diabetes. Many cancers are hormone related. Estrogen dominance may be accountable for breast, prostate, cervix, endometrial, uterine, and ovarian cancer as well as fibroids. Estrogen deficiency can also cause bladder and urinary tract infections, especially in menopausal women.

Progesterone deficiency can cause cancer as well, including uterine cancer and fibroids. The thicker the lining of the uterus, the higher the chances of cancer are. Natural progesterone cream can help to reduce the lining of the uterine wall and eliminate fibroids in as little as two months; so the cream is not something that needs to be taken forever.

Maintaining a healthy liver is also extremely important to managing uterine fibroids because it is responsible for eliminating toxins from the body. A healthy liver converts the strongest estrogen to "safe estrogen". Remember that certain medications including birth control pills, fertility drugs, and hormone replacement therapy can also create a state of estrogen dominance. Excess estrogen can be promoted by liver congestion, bowel toxicity, stress, hypothyroidism, inflammation, and many of the estrogens below.

Supplementing with DIM can help reduce the steady climb of estrogen. It has been reported that DIM or diindolylmethane can reduce estrogen buildup. It does this by converting bad estrogen into good estrogen by-products. It is also said to help reduce a swollen prostate.

Many researchers also attribute the high incidence of cancers to the presence of environmental estrogens in our food and products today. Phytoestrogens are plant-derived xenoestrogens and are consumed by eating phytoestrogenic plants. They imitate estrogen, but are not generated within the endocrine system; Phytoestrogens can be either synthetic (man-made) or natural chemical compounds.

Here are some examples of hormones, food or toxins that may

alter balance:

Xenoestrogens: artificial scents, air fresheners, food additives, preservatives, commercially raised poultry and cattle, household cleaners, detergents, car exhaust and indoor toxins, personal care products (shampoos, lotions, perfumes, makeup, deodorants), oral contraceptives, prescription drugs, paints, lacquers and solvents, pesticides, herbicides, fertilizers, Styrofoam products, plant estrogens (soy, flaxseed), plastics, canned foods, GMOs and plastic food wrap.

Naturally Estrogenic: alcohol, alfalfa, anise seed, apples, barley, beets, black-eyed peas, blue/black cohosh, cherries, chickpeas, clover, cucumbers, dairy, dates, dong quai, eggs, eggplant, fennel, flaxseed, flour, garlic, hops, lavender, licorice, meat, oats, olive oil, olives, papaya, parsley, peas, peppers, plums, pomegranates, poppy seed, potatoes, pumpkin, red beans, red clover, rhodiola, rose root, rhubarb, rice, sage, saw palmetto, sesame seeds, soybean, sprouts, sugar, sunflower seeds, tea tree oil, tomatoes, wheat, white rice., soy, canola, safflower and corn oil.

Foods That Inhibit Estrogen: artichoke, asparagus, avocados, berries, brazil nuts, broccoli, buckwheat, cabbage, celery, citrus fruits (except apples, cherries, dates, pomegranates), figs, garlic, grapes, green beans, green tea, melons, nuts, onions, pears, pineapples, seaweed, squash, tapioca, white flour, white rice.

Balancing Hormones: Moringa, carrots, chia seeds, coconut oil, cod liver oil, Diindolylmethane (DIM), false unicorn, gelatin, kelp, maca root, magnesium, olive leaf extract, parsley, quinoa, red raspberry, Vitamin D, flaxseed oil*.

Increases Progesterone: beta carotene, chaste berry, dill, legumes, oregano, seeds, sweet potato, thyme, turmeric, vegetables, Vitamin B6, C & E, L-arginine, wild yam. There are also natural progesterone creams.

*A note about flaxseed oil. "Research shows that adding flax oil to foods rich in sulfated amino acids, such as cultured dairy products (i.e., cottage cheese), vegetables of the cabbage family... helps the essential fatty acids become incorporated into cell membranes." In fact, The Budwig Center has a flaxseed oil and cottage cheese protocol that has been reported by their patients to eliminate tumors, degenerative diseases, balance hormones, cure Arthritis, Asthma, Fibromyalgia, Diabetes, Blood Pressure, Multiple Sclerosis, Heart Disease, Psoriasis, Eczema, Acne and more.

What about Menopause?

The average age that women go through menopause is about 51. Menopause can really cause havoc on one's body and it's not always the easiest thing to go through. Again, it is recommended that you be evaluated by your physician before self-prescribing for hormone-related problems.

Here are some symptoms of menopause:

Hot flashes, night sweats (Consider using: Cod Liver Oil, Red Clover Tea)

Loss of libido (Maca root)

Allergic Reactions

Food sensitivities such as gluten (Use only organic wheat)

Fatigue

Hair loss (Castor Oil)

Weight gain (Moringa)

Bloating, indigestion

Anxiety, depression (Brewer's Yeast)

Mood swings

Sleep disorders (Moringa)

Memory lapses (Cod Liver Oil)

Dizziness

Osteoporosis (Cod Liver Oil)

Uterine lining thickening, fibroids (Natural progesterone)

An interesting study from 2011 entitled: Estrogenic botanical supplements, health-related quality of life, fatigue, and hormone-related symptoms in breast cancer survivors: a HEAL study reported the following conclusions:

- Flaxseed oil users were more likely to have a better mental health summary score.

- Ginseng users were more likely to report severe fatigue and several hormone-related symptoms.

- Red clover users were less likely to report weight gain, night sweats, and difficulty concentrating.

- Alfalfa users were less likely to experience sleep

interruption.

- Dehydroepiandrosterone users were less likely to have hot flashes.

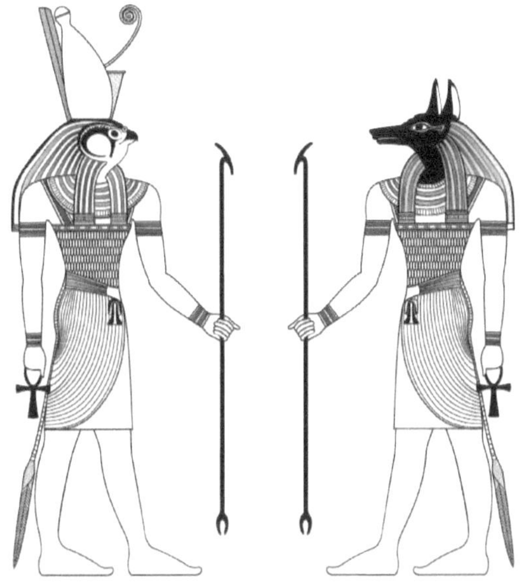

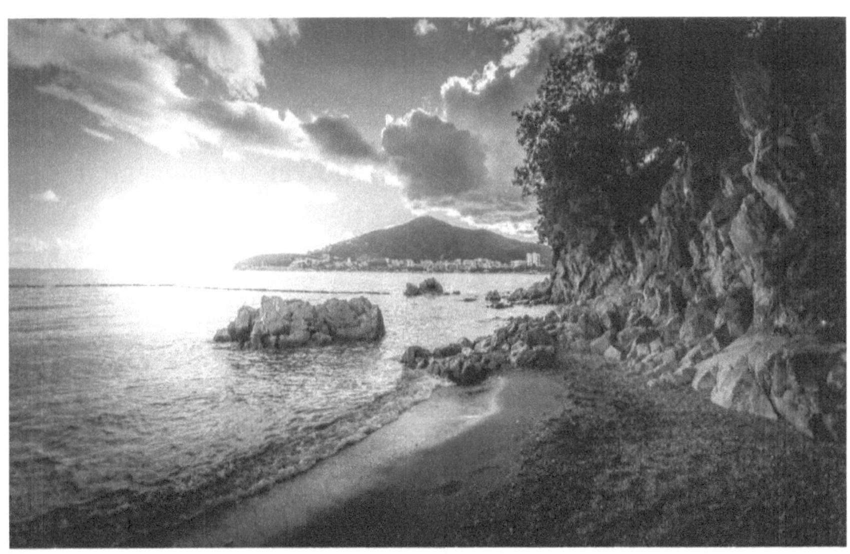

FOREVER LIVING PRODUCT

FOREVER CALCIUM®

Science has shown that as we age our ability to absorb calcium reduces. In fact, some reports indicate that our ability to absorb calcium from our diet declines by 60% from childhood to adulthood. What can you do to promote healthy bones and teeth? New & Improved Forever Calcium® provides the clinically proven quantities of Calcium, Magnesium, Zinc, Manganese, Copper and the Vitamin C & D to help maintain proper bone structure and function.

You depend on the strength of your body every day, and it starts from the inside out. Forever's new form of calcium, Di-Calcium malate, is most effective at promoting optimum bone building since it stays in the bloodstream longer and does not interfere with the natural pH balance in the stomach. Additionally, our proprietary mineral blend is smaller and more absorbable than our previous formula.

New & Improved Forever Calcium® uses superior forms of calcium and other patented high-performance minerals to ensure maximum absorption and bioavailability. To combat our declining ability to absorb calcium as we age, a comprehensive supplement is vital to help protect against bone loss. Forever Calcium® can help you feel assured that you are relying on the highest quality ingredients to support your health.

* Provides Calcium, Magnesium, Zinc, Manganese, Copper and the Vitamin C & D

* Ensure maximum absorption and bioavailability.

FOREVER ABSORBENT-C®

Daily vitamin C has long been associated with good health. Science now provides us with a whole list of benefits derived from this most famous of all vitamins:

It is a powerful antioxidant, forming part of the body's defense system against the harmful effects of free radicals.

It is a beneficial supplement for the skin, as it supports the formation of intercellular collagen

It is necessary for the maintenance of healthy connective tissue.

Vitamin C is water soluble and is secreted from the body. Since humans are among the few animals that are unable to make their own vitamin C, we must, therefore, get it from our food, drinks, and supplements, such as Forever Absorbent-C®.

The need for adequate levels of vitamin C is very evident. Science reports that one cigarette destroys 25mg of vitamin C.

Stress, medication and environmental factors all heavily deplete the body of this vitamin. A deficiency can result in broken capillaries and bleeding gums.

Forever Absorbent-C® with Oat Bran is an outstanding nutritional supplement. It combines two vital nutrients into one convenient product. The bonded matrix composition is a unique delivery system combining 500 mg of oat bran with the full 60 mg of Vitamin C in each tablet.

A daily intake of Forever® Absorbent-C® is highly recommended for good health.

Oat bran aids absorption of vitamin C

Powerful antioxidant

Promotes healthy skin

FOREVER IMMUBLEND®

Forever ImmuBlend™ is designed to support immune system function by addressing all aspects of the immune system from its first line of defense to its last. Each ingredient in our proprietary blend is specifically chosen for the crucial role it plays in supporting your body's immune system function. It helps the body's biological defense system to operate at peak performance so you can carry on your daily routine without any cares.

Our immune-enhancing nutrient blend includes the power of lactoferrin, maitake and shiitake mushrooms, along with Vitamin C & D and zinc for that extra support your body needs.

Each of these key ingredients contributes to your body's well-being:

Fructooligosaccharides – promote healthy levels of probiotic bacteria in the digestive system.

Lactoferrin – supports immune cell production and helps maintain optimum levels of beneficial bacteria in the intestines

Maitake & Shiitake Mushrooms – support immune cell production and cardiovascular function •Vitamin D – strengthens immune cells

Vitamin C –fights free radicals

Zinc – fights free radicals and supports immune cell production

This exclusive formula addresses all aspects of immune system function, providing both foundational nutrients required for a healthy immune system and natural botanicals that work synergistically to support immune function.

Supports all aspects of immune system function

Provides a variety of nutrients to support immune system activity

Fights free radicals

FOREVER KIDS®

Give your kids the nutrients they need each day with Forever Kids® Chewable Multivitamins. These fun and delicious multivitamins provide both adults and growing kids ages two and older with the vital vitamins, minerals, iron and phytonutrients they may be lacking.

Iron is a new addition to Forever Kids for its role in immune support and cognitive development. Iron, a commonly deficient nutrient, also supports overall health.

Phytonutrients are highly desirable plant nutrients found in vegetables and fruits. Our new and improved formula has more phytonutrients from a new, improved blend of fruits and vegetables. The result is a multivitamin that tastes great, is fun to eat and complements the range of other supplements that Forever Living offers!

Formulated without artificial colors or preservatives, the phytonutrient base is taken from such nutritious foods as carrots, beets, broccoli, spinach, blueberries, apples, cranberries, tomatoes, and strawberries. You and your kids will love the natural grape flavor, and you'll love the peace of mind!

No artificial colors or preservatives.

Chewable tablets.

Phytonutrient base taken from the finest raw foods, including broccoli, spinach, beets, and carrots.

FOREVER DAILY®

Forever Daily® is a revolutionary nutrient delivery system designed in combination with Forever Living's proprietary aloe oligosaccharide (AOS) complex. Forever Daily® with AOS delivers a perfectly balanced blend of 55 nutrients, including essential vitamins and minerals, providing more efficient absorption and in the case of minerals, targeting specific body systems.

Additionally, Forever Daily's comprehensive nutritional program delivers optimal amounts of important natural phytonutrients, bioflavonoids, cutting-edge antioxidants with molecular-technology, and a proprietary blend of fruits and vegetables to ensure your body receives all the essential.

This unique formula is designed to nourish and protect our bodies by filling the nutrient gaps in our everyday diet and provide optimal health and vitality.

* Blend of 55 nutrients, including essential vitamins and minerals.

* Nourishes and protects our bodies.

FOREVER A-BETA-CARE®

Forever A-Beta-CarE® is an essential formula combining vitamins A (from beta-carotene) and E, plus the antioxidant mineral Selenium. Antioxidants are vital in the fight against free radicals (chemical molecules that arise from pollutants in the body and damage healthy cells).

Vitamin A plays an important role in vision, bone growth, reproduction, and cell division. It helps maintain the surface linings of the eyes and the respiratory, urinary, and intestinal tracts. Forever A-Beta-CarE® is a specially formulated dietary supplement that supplies vitamin A to the body from beta-carotene. The body converts beta-carotene to vitamin A in the small intestine during digestion or when it is needed, leaving a low risk of vitamin A overdose (which can be toxic when taken alone in large doses). Beta-carotene is also a recognized antioxidant, making it an ideal companion for vitamin E and Selenium.

Vitamin E, a fat-soluble vitamin, is an excellent supplement for healthy skin. It also protects vitamin A and essential fatty acids from oxidation in the body cells and prevents the breakdown of body tissues.

Selenium is a trace mineral and is one of the most powerful antioxidant nutrients known to work synergistically with both vitamin E and beta-carotene. It is beneficial in maintaining healthy skin, hair and good eyesight. Recent research shows that Selenium is especially important to men's health.

This combination of nutrients, available all in one convenient product, is one of the most important complements to good health.

FOREVER B12 PLUS®

An excellent combination of essential nutrients, Forever B12 Plus® combines Vitamin B12 with Folic Acid utilizing a time-release formula to help make possible metabolic processes - including cell division, DNA synthesis, red blood cell production, and proper nerve function.

Vitamin B12, or Cyanocobalamin, was first discovered in 1948 as a nutritional factor that is vital for red blood cell production. B12 also works with folic acid to maintain healthy homocysteine levels in the body.

Perform this first act of love for your baby! Vitamin B12 deficiency also means deficiency in folic acid, which is critical to the fetus during the first three months of pregnancy, also making it beneficial to women wishing to conceive.

This supplement is extremely safe, as both components are tolerated in large amounts. It is also essential to a vegetarian or vegan diet, as B12 is normally obtained from animal sources.

Enjoy the benefits of Vitamin B12 and folic acid together, in a formula exclusively designed to complement the rest of our supplement range!

Helps maintain healthy homocysteine levels

Extremely safe, even in large amounts

Supplements of vitamin B12 and folic acid should be taken together.

VIT♂LIZE™ MEN'S

Although the exact age may vary, prostate health eventually becomes an important issue for all men. Vit♂lize™ Men's Vitality Supplement contains all of the power of Forever Pr♂6®, but now also includes more nutrients, more bioavailable nutrient forms and more powerful botanicals.

Vit♂lize™, combined with a healthy diet and exercise, offers a natural solution to support prostate health. This unique, comprehensive formulation supplies a highly effective blend of potent herbs, vitamins, minerals, and antioxidants to help maintain normal urinary flow, promote healthy testicular function, and encourage optimal prostate health.

Proprietary Botanical Blend

Vit♂lize™ is formulated with a proprietary blend of botanicals including saw palmetto, pygeum and pumpkin seed. Each of these botanicals has been used for centuries to support prostate health.

Exclusive Nutrient Blend

Vit♂lize™ also includes a blend of nutrients specifically designed and balanced to support men's health and promote healthy prostate function. Vitamin C, D, E, and B6 are all essential for a healthy prostate. These vitamins have been combined with the minerals selenium and zinc, which have been found to play a critical role in prostate health. Quercetin and lycopene have also been added in levels that are properly balanced with these critical nutrients to provide complete prostate support.

New & Improved

In addition to vitamin E, selenium and lycopene from the original Forever Pr♂6®, Vitamin C, D and B6 have been added in combination with zinc and quercetin. Vitamin C, D, and B6 are all essential for prostate health and are required for the production of hormones.

A proprietary botanical blend including saw palmetto, pygeum and pumpkin seed

Proper nutrient balance for complete prostate support

Provides polyphenols equivalent to eating an entire pomegranate fruit.

FOREVER IMMUBLEND®

Forever ImmuBlend™ is designed to support immune system function by addressing all aspects of the immune system from its first line of defense to its last. Each ingredient in our proprietary blend is specifically chosen for the crucial role it plays in supporting your body's immune system function. It helps the body's biological defense system to operate at peak performance so you can carry on your daily routine without any cares.

Our immune-enhancing nutrient blend includes the power of lactoferrin, maitake and shiitake mushrooms, along with Vitamin C & D and zinc for that extra support your body needs. Each of these key ingredients contributes to your body's well-being:

Fructooligosaccharides – promote healthy levels of probiotic bacteria in the digestive system.

Lactoferrin – supports immune cell production and helps maintain optimum levels of beneficial bacteria in the intestines

Maitake & Shiitake Mushrooms – support immune cell production and cardiovascular function •Vitamin D – strengthens immune cells

Vitamin C –fights free radicals

Zinc – fights free radicals and supports immune cell production

This exclusive formula addresses all aspects of immune system function, providing both foundational nutrients required for a healthy immune system and natural botanicals that work synergistically to support immune function.

Supports all aspects of immune system function

Provides a variety of nutrients to support immune system activity

Fights free radicals.

FOREVER ARCTIC SEA®

New and improved Forever Arctic Sea® now contains a proprietary blend of DHA-rich Calamari Oil, ultra-pure Omega-3 Fish Oil, and High Oleic Olive Oil. This unique blend is exclusive to Forever Living and provides not only 33% more DHA per day, but creates the perfect balance of DHA and EPA for optimal health and wellness.

The Critical Omega-3: Omega-6 Balance

There is an important balance that most people do not fully understand when it comes to Omegas. Historically, nutritionally balanced diets contained a healthy ratio of Omegas as 1:1 up to 1:4 DHA: EPA. Unfortunately, many diets include unhealthy levels of Omega-6's which are traditionally derived from fried foods, vegetable oils, fake butter products, grain-fed animal fat and other modern convenience and processed foods. In addition, many diets are low in fish and Omega-3 consumption, which creates an unhealthy ratio of Omega-6: Omega-3 as high as 30:1! The key to getting back to a healthy ratio of DHA: EPA is increasing Omega-3 consumption and reducing Omega-6 intake.

Forever Arctic Sea® has been improved to not only increase the total amount of Omega-3's you get per serving but also has significantly increased the amount of DHA per dose. DHA Omega-3 is naturally found throughout the body and is most abundant in the brain, eyes, and heart. Just as calcium is essential for building strong bones, DHA ensures that the cells in the brain, retina, heart and other parts of the nervous system develop and function properly through all stages of life. Additionally, DHA intake has been associated with a decreased risk of mental decline associated with aging. No other fatty acid demonstrates this relationship.

Custom Omega-3 ratio to mimic a diet rich in seafood

All-natural citrus flavor for a pleasant aroma and minimal fishy flavor

Ocean friendly and responsibly sourced • Pure source of EPA and DHA.

FOREVER GARLIC-THYME®

The dietary use of garlic and thyme has been traced back thousands of years. An Egyptian papyrus dating from 1,500BC listed 22 healthy uses for garlic. Today, we are starting to understand how they work.

Garlic and thyme, the two powerful antioxidants found in Forever Garlic-Thyme®, combine to create a great tool in maintaining good health. When garlic is cut or crushed, enzymes react to produce a powerful immune-enhancing agent. Studies have shown that garlic's other ingredients help the metabolism convert fats to energy and protect the body against free radicals.

Thyme contains saponins and other beneficial antioxidant substances.

Powerful antioxidant.

Odorless, soft gel capsule.

Helps protect the body against free radicals.

Helps support the conversion of fats to energy.

NATURE-MIN®

Your body can benefit from nutrients locked deep in an ancient seabed because four percent of our body weight is comprised of these minerals. Since our bodies can't manufacture minerals, we have to obtain them from our food or supplementation.

Forever Nature-Min® is an advanced, multi-mineral formula using new bio-available forms of minerals for maximum absorption. It provides minerals and traces minerals in a perfectly balanced ratio for maximum efficiency. Using a mineral base of natural seabed deposits, Nature-Min provides most of the key minerals found in the human body.

Minerals in the body perform three functions:

1. Some, like calcium, phosphorus, and magnesium, are constituents of the bones and teeth.

2. Others are soluble salts that help to control the composition of body fluids and cells.

3. Minerals, such as iron and hemoglobin, perform other vital tasks. They work with enzymes and proteins, which are necessary for releasing and utilizing energy.

Forever Nature-Min® is an excellent way to ensure that your body is getting the minerals and trace minerals it needs to meet the demands of a healthy, balanced lifestyle.

Contains trace minerals from natural sea bed deposit.

A perfect blend of minerals in each tablet.

Minerals play many roles in the human body, from regulating fluid balance to activating genes and hormones.

Supplements That Prevent Aging

When explorers first arrived in the new world, rumors abounded of a mythical fountain whose water was said to give one eternal youth. Though many hopeful searchers spent their lives in pursuit of this fantasy, in the end, they became old and past quietly into history. Today, rumors have returned about a "fountain of youth", but this time they aren't based on myth, but come from solid scientific research.

As science digs deeper and deeper into genetic research, more and more evidence emerges that humans do not have to age as they do. Research suggests that humans can essentially live forever given the proper conditions. Though science has many years ahead of it before it can truly stop the aging process, several nutritional supplements that prevent aging have been discovered. New discoveries arrive almost daily lending credibility to the effectiveness of certain supplements in slowing the aging process and anyone interested in staying young and healthy should investigate the findings. Here are a few of the best supplements available today to combat aging.

CoQ10 (Coenzyme Q10)

This is an enzyme that has numerous beneficial effects on the body. It is a powerful antioxidant that is especially effective in preventing heart disease. CoQ10 acts on every cell in the body and aid in energy production and cell rejuvenation. Evidence suggests that this enzyme is also very effective against breast cancer.

Resveratrol

Resveratrol is the chemical upon which scientists are staking their hopes for a true anti-aging drug. This is the age preventing chemical found in red wine, which has gotten so much press over the years as an antioxidant, heart saver and cancer fighter. Resveratrol is available in pill and contrary to popular belief, you would have to drink much more red wine than your body could tolerate in order to derive the anti-aging and health benefits of Resveratrol anyway.

Vitamin E

This is perhaps one of the first supplements giving credit for preventing aging. It consists of a number of powerful antioxidant compounds that aid in cell repair and have been proven to prevent and fight cancer. Though supplementation of vitamin E is recommended, care must be taken since high levels of vitamin E can be toxic.

Vitamin C

Most people have heard of vitamin C in its role in the prevention of the common cold. though that has recently been disputed, its role as an all-around age preventing supplement is gaining momentum. It is another antioxidant that plays a role in cellular repair throughout the body. Vitamin C is water soluble and therefore is virtually impossible to take too much. Though available in supplement form, it is best when found in fresh fruits and vegetables.

Ease of Taking Supplements

Supplements by design are one of the easiest things that you can do to slow down the aging process. And many of these supplements not only help reverse the aesthetic effects of aging, but also the biological effects that aging has on organ systems and overall health.

This small list is just a drop in the ocean of age preventing supplements available today. Some of these supplements have scientifically proven track records while others are still being investigated.

Safety of Supplements

Consumers should research supplements before taking them to ensure they are right for their particular situation. If in doubt, individuals should check with their doctors prior to beginning a supplement regimen. Some supplements can interfere with medications that you may be taking, minimizing their effects or rendering them useless. It is especially important to check with your doctor before taking any type of supplement if you have a major health issue.

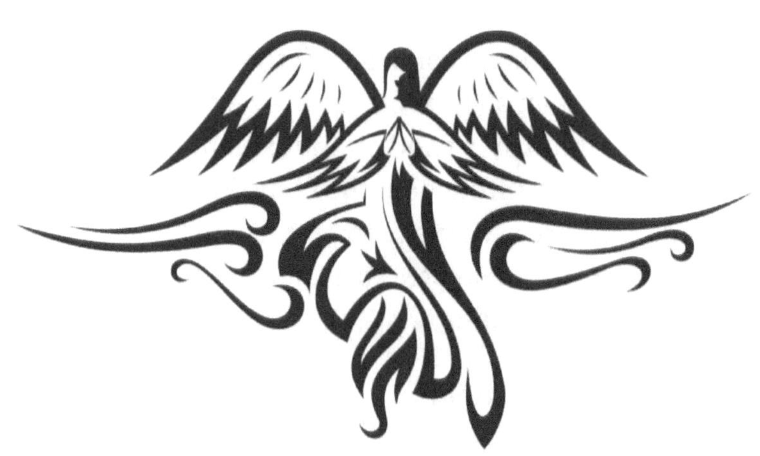

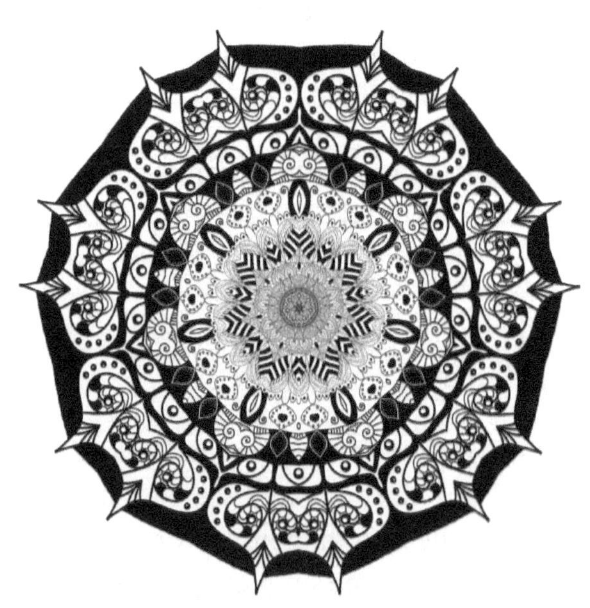

PROTECT YOURSELF FROM FREE RADICAL DAMAGE

BETA-CAROTENE, for example, is one voracious phytochemical found in raw yellow and orange fruit and other vegetables. These raw foods have proven to be beneficial in reducing damage to cells caused by free radicals. Free radicals work to damage cells, fueling the aging process through cell mutation and cell death. One molecule of beta-carotene can kill up to one thousand free radicals.

Research is also mounting on alpha lipoic acid. As an antioxidant, alpha lipoic acid is very powerful. For the past thirty years throughout Europe, it has been used to stabilize blood sugar in treating diabetes

USE RAW AND WHOLE FOODS TO REVITALIZE HEALTH

Diet is one of the best ways to maintain our youth or reverse the aging process. The nutrients in raw and whole foods, accompanied with various supplements, are the chemical elements used by the body to ward off disease and maintain health. The combinations of deficiencies of vital nutrients, toxicity from the environment, and a poor diet contributes to disease. Eating whole and raw foods may be issues for some people, but for those who can digest whole foods, the benefits are enormous.

People are constantly trying to get life from lifeless food. All enzymes are destroyed by heat, diminishing the life force in food. Enzymes are wiped out when temperatures start to reach 118 degrees. Once 140 degrees is reached, enzymes are lost. Our body produces certain enzymes, but the burden upon our systems would be greatly lessened with a plentiful supply from our diet. The body does its best but will eventually fall short without a replenishing supply.

FEED YOUR GLANDS TO STAY YOUNG

When the diet is deficient in a particular chemical element required by a specific organ or gland, our bodies will be vulnerable to disease. We are only as young as our glands. Glands need whole foods such as nuts, seeds, sprouts, egg yolk, and sardines (with the bones), hard cheese, whole grains and algae. Nuts and seeds are among our most complete foods. They contain hormone value for both the male and female glands. They are small but mighty, loaded with glandular elements, vitamins, minerals and proteins. Almonds are the king of nuts and sesame seeds are the king of seeds. However, sick people do not handle cold proteins well. For this reason, nut and seed drinks, butter, meals and soy milk powders are recommended. Sprouts contain auxins, a substance which promotes plant growth. A diet high in sprouts will provide the auxins for cell stimulation and life force. People from cultures whose diets are plentiful in sprouts typically retain their youthfulness and vigor well into their advanced years.

THE HIDDEN HEALTH BENEFITS OF FIBER

Fiber is another whole food highly recommended for stimulating peristalsis and moving food along our intestines. Studies show that when bile acids are retained by fiber, the body absorbs less cholesterol. There is growing evidence that fiber in the diet will lower your blood fats and may protect against degenerative diseases such as cancer, atherosclerosis and diabetes. In addition, case studies show that a patient's blood sugar is not as high following a meal of high fiber as compared to a meal of processed low fiber food. Blood sugar is lowered when the fiber slows down and smooths out the absorption of sugars from the intestine.

JUICING: GREAT SOURCE FOR NUTRIENTS AND ENZYMES

Juicing is another excellent source for supplying the body with live foods rich in nutrients. If you are tired, sluggish or stressed, fresh juice will give you a boost. Though it may be better to eat the whole plant, juicing is the next best thing for those who have difficulty digesting whole foods, raw vegetables and citrus fruits. Also, the amount one is able to consume in a day may be an issue. Fruit juice is a great source of vitamins and vegetable juice is higher in the chemical elements which build and tone our bodies.

USE ORGANIC SODIUM TO STAY YOUTHFUL

Organic sodium is one of our "youth elements". It is found in our joints, ligaments and our stomachs. If we want to stay youthful and pliable, we need organic sodium. The highest form is found in whey powder, while other sources are goat milk, celery, okra, most fruits except for citrus, dark leafy vegetables, fish, black olives, lentils, dulse, barely and sesame seeds. Organic sodium keeps calcium in solution, preventing osteoarthritis and cataracts. This beneficial sodium should not be confused with table salts, which leach the good organic sodium from our bodies.

Another consideration to maintain our youth is to keep our bodies alkaline. Our blood pH is highly alkaline: twenty percent acid and eighty percent alkaline. For optimum health, our diet should match our blood balance. Organs and glands need alkaline secretions. Essentially, all vegetables and fruit are alkaline with a few exceptions. Citrus fruit is acid, although lemons have an alkaline ash. All starch and protein are acid forming foods. Dairy products are for the most part acidic. However, yogurt, kefir, buttermilk, raw milk, whey and acidophilus culture are considered alkaline.

We should also eat a variety of fruits and vegetables when they are in season and plentiful - all colors of the rainbow. Fruit is natures' cleanser and meant to be eaten in more abundance following a long winter season of heavy food. Chlorophyll, the green juice found in vegetables and plants has the ability to clean and heal, inside and out. When it comes to our overall well-being and state of health, we must look to the source from which the elements in our bodies come. Foods in their natural state can heal us, feed us and keep us forever young.

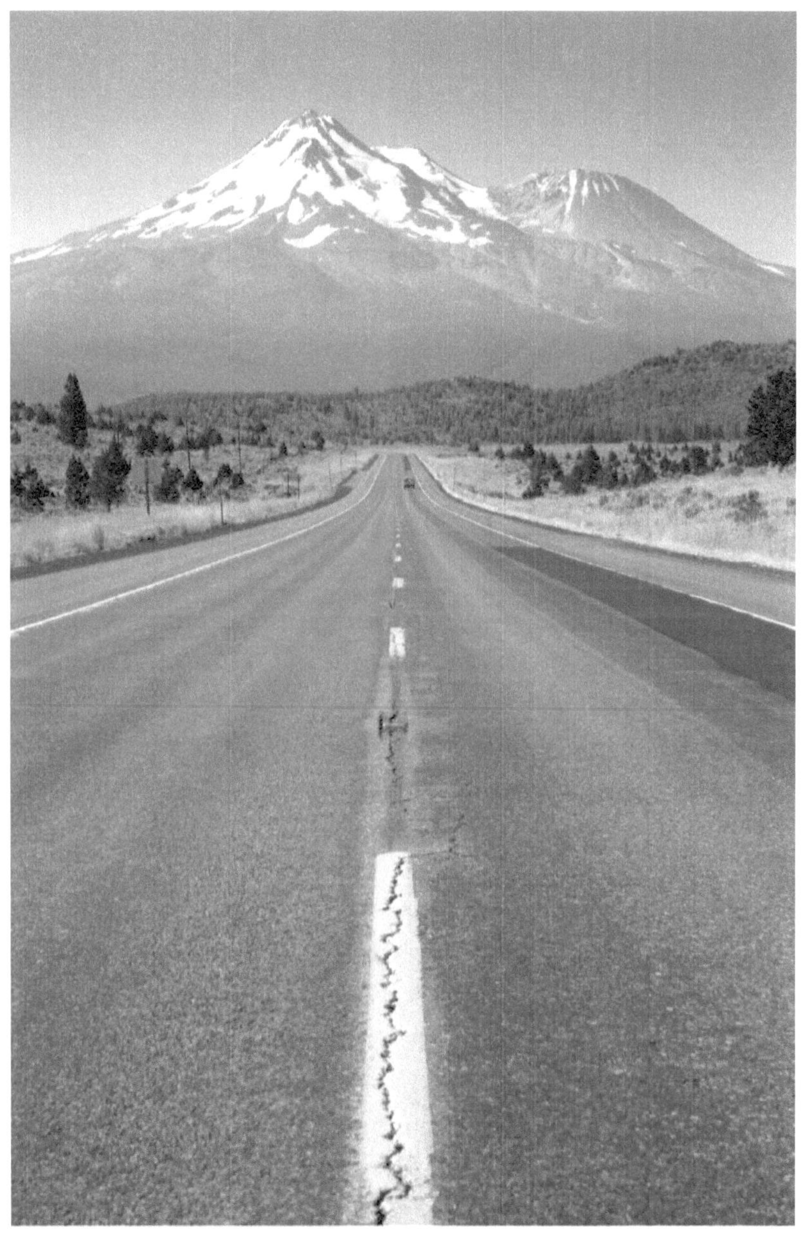

BILLIE WOODARD AND TWIN SISTER, ZURIA IN HOLLOW EARTH

BILLIE FAYE WOODARD and his twin sister, Zuria, were born in the Inner Earth, and brought to the outer Earth on September 18, 1951. They were both born with exceptional abilities, including the ability to speak an ancient Lemurian language. Both Billie and his sister were born with both male and female organs, and were hermaphrodites, but over the years Billie has become more masculine and today he has become very strong and speaks with a masculine voice.

His exceptional abilities and intelligence led him to a rapid rise in the military, and during the late 1960s, he rose to the rank of Colonel and became the base commander of Area 51. During his time there, he took a shuttle craft from the base to visit his parents in the Inner Earth. He is in touch with his parents now and visits the Inner Earth frequently.

In these interviews, I talk with Billie Faye and his father Zorra from the Hollow Earth, who speaks through Billie. Zorra gives important messages to humanity from the Inner Earth and the beautiful bright future for all of us!

They were born with exceptional abilities. Billie can remember their parents talking to them as babies. Soon after their birth, their Hollow Earth parents told them they would not be living with them any longer. They were taken to Wichita Falls, Texas and put in a litter barrel garbage container in a park where a passing park attendant and a police officer heard them crying. They were retrieved and put in an orphanage and about 5 years later were adopted by a US Air Force Colonel Woodard, his wife and two sons. Billie's adoptive parents were both of American Indian descent, the mother an Apache, and adoptive father, a Cherokee. Billie's adoptive mother died this year and was cremated in a sacred Apache burial ritual which Billie was able to attend. The adoptive father is still living, but not doing too well in health.

At the age of five, Billie remembers talking to his sister when they were at a restaurant with their adopted parents and a nearby man exclaimed with great surprise to their parents, "Do you know what your children are saying over there, in their communication? Do you know that your children are talking to each other in an extinct language? I am a professor of ancient languages at the University of Texas (at Austin) and your children are speaking to each other in the extinct Lemurian language!"

Among the unusual characteristics, Billie and his sister had was that they were born with both male and female organs. They were, in fact, hermaphrodites, but with the years Billie has become more masculine. Today Billie speaks in a deep masculine voice, and has become quite strong. Regrettably, Billie admits that the step father was a pedophile that molested

Billie at a very young age on a regular basis, and invited one of the brothers to molest also until Billie told some of his classmates at school at the age of 10. The step father would put sleeping pills in his wife's drink at meal time so she would go to sleep while he went up into Billie's attic room to molest Billie, where Billie was kept locked up most of the time. When the step-father heard that the word had gotten out at school, he immediately stopped molesting Billie and took Billie to the US Air Force base hospital and had Billie's vagina sealed and the ovaries and uterus removed. With the female organs removed, Billie became only male. The step father then made Billie dress in male clothing. For this molestation, the step-father spent some time in jail and later the Air Force removed Billie from that family and was placed with another Indian family near Apache Junction, Arizona.

Billie's sister was separated from them at the age of six. It happened when they were both taken to a base where they were given all kinds of tests on their exceptional abilities. At one point, Billie decided no more tests were bearable, and so with just mind control, Billie created havoc with the test readings. Soon after this, Billie's adoptive father sold Billie's sister to another Air Force Sergeant for $1 million dollars.

The military told them that the sister later had died in the tests that they had given her, but they later learned that she hadn't died, but was taken to an underground base for more testing, and soon after was taken to our Hollow Earth by a Hollow Earth flying saucer that rescued her from her military captors.

Soon after the adopted father had gotten out of jail, Billie was coming home from a Scout activity with a friend, and as they neared their home in the countryside, Billie wanted to take a short cut through a corn field, but the friend insisted on continuing on the road for fear of walking through the cornstalks. After passing through the corn field, Billie was coming close to home when a man in uniform shouted into his mobile phone, "We have found Billie! Call off the search!"

Billie wondered what was going on. The parents wanted to know where Billie had been for the past six months, and Billie replied, "What do you mean? I just came home from Scouts with my friend." The friend that lived next door had rushed over at the commotion and remarked, "But that was six months ago!"

So the step-father took Billie in to the military base, and an hypnotic session was run to help recall what had happened in the missing time.

With the help of the hypnotic regression, Billie recalled what had happened that late summer evening when coming home with the friend from the Scout activity. As Billie had walked through the corn field, Billie had noticed a bright star that seemed to get brighter and brighter until a round metallic shape was visible. When it got closer, Billie could see that it was about 150 feet in diameter and looked like a flying saucer space craft. A strange, but soothing, soft angelic music was coming from it and a pleasant voice asked, "Billie, would you like to take a journey with us on our ship?" Billie replied that that would be fun, and immediately began floating up in the air towards the ship and was taken aboard.

The flying saucer occupants were very friendly, but very large in stature. There were several crew members, but a man and a woman were attending to Billie. The woman was about 10 feet tall and the man about 13 feet tall. Billie remarked to them that they were very tall and large people. They said that Billie was a very perceptive person and asked how Billie was doing in geography at school. Billie let them know that straight "A's" were received in school, and even recognized the places they were flying over. As they would fly over each state's capital on the way north, Billie recognized and named off the different state flags. As they reached Canada, where Billie had been to Calgary at one time during the Calgary Rodeo Stampede with a step-brother, Billie recognized the city.

The flying saucer then flew up over the Arctic and Billie was asked about what was seen and where they were. Billie said there was ice and snow but didn't know where they were. They told Billie they were flying over northern Canada and soon they were out over the Arctic Ocean covered with ice floes. The craft then flew through a big hole in the Arctic Ocean into the interior of the earth where they could see an interior sun shining and many cities on the interior surface of the planet. There Billie lived with them for six months. While there, Billie met many people that had disappeared from the surface of the Earth, such as pilots lost in the Bermuda triangle. They were now large in stature. After living in the earth for a time as result of the less gravity there, Billie says this allows people living there to grow larger in stature. There, Billie also met his sister again, who told Billie that in six months time Billie would be sent back to the surface world. After the six months stay in the Hollow Earth, Billie was returned to Texas and was left in the corn field with no recollection of the trip.

The Air Force later removed Billie from the Woodard family at age 13 and he was adopted by the Henderson family, but with no change of name, at which time they lived near Apache Junction, Arizona. Henderson worked for the military but was not a military man. At that time, Billie attended the Apache

Reservation school by school bus and graduated from High School on the Apache Reservation in their advanced gifted program at an early age.

After Billie graduated from High School, and after waiting a couple of years, the new step father signed an approval for Billie to join the Air Force. So after Basic Training of 8 weeks, and then advanced training for 6 weeks, Billie signed an agreement to be stationed in Hawaii, but instead was taken to the Pentagon and told that the next assignment was a top secret facility in the Nevada desert known as Area 51, and that the current rank of Lieutenant was not sufficient for that assignment and so he was advanced to field commission of Colonel.

On the way to Area 51, they boarded a four engine prop plane at Nellis Air Force Base near Las Vegas, Nevada. It was morning when they boarded the airplane and Billie noticed that all the windows were blackened out so they couldn't see out. A short time later they landed and got out of the airplane at Area 51. To Billie, it looked like night time. Billie remarked as to why it was so dark and why they could see no stars. Billie was told they were inside a mountain. They boarded a staff car and soon started down a 45 degree angle incline which was somewhat alarming. Soon the car reached another level and Billie was told to get out and go into a building and take off all clothes. Soon a pink mist filled the room in some kind of decontamination routine.

With a new set of clothes on, they took the vehicle down another steep incline to another level far beneath the previous level and were told to go into another building where a blue mist this time filled the room for another type of decontamination. Billie was given a new uniform that had a triangle logo with the numbers 51 on it. Outside the patch was another circle with the words, "Black Project" and on the bottom of the circle the words, "Top Secret."

They then got into an elevator and went down to another level. The elevator descended so rapidly that they were almost weightless. It soon slowed down and stopped and when the elevator doors opened, they were looking at a nice little underground town with people walking here and there. It is located on the 10th level. It looked as bright as daylight just like a little town on the surface world, except they couldn't see very far. There was a sun-like orb in the sky and above that was pitch black. Billie's living quarters were on this 10th level.

Billie was then taken to an assigned office on the 6th level in Archives and relieved the previous on-duty officer, who remarked that he was happy to be leaving. Billie asked him, "Why?", but he just shrugged and said that he had had enough. He said, "You'll find out soon enough why I just want to get out of here and why am glad to be leaving." Billie sat down at the desk and looked through the files and folders on the desk. The files and folders were classified documentation the military has gathered over the years on Our Hollow Earth. Among the documents, Billie was able to study a 35 page document on Admiral Richard E. Byrd's journeys to Our Hollow Earth through both the north and south polar openings. Billie distinctly remembers reading the exact coordinates of the north polar opening that leads into Our Hollow Earth. A day later a higher ranking officer came and said, "Your presence is requested on a lower level. You were asked for by name."

Billie was then taken to still another lower level that opened into a tunnel where a shuttle train waited. The new attendants who greeted Billie were very tall, one was male and the other was female. They seemed to be giants compared to Billie's own height of 5' 11". They were similar to those that had taken Billie on the flying saucer at age 12. They greeted Billie pleasantly in English and invited Billie to step aboard the shuttle train and was asked to strap in. When Billie asked where they would be going, they said, "Telos," a sacred Lemurian city beneath Mt. Shasta, California where Billie met their great High Priest leader, Adama and his wife, Raia and was given a tour of their underground city.

For the next 11 and half years, Billie journeyed three times to our Hollow Earth in shuttle craft through the underground tunnels, and subsequently also to many other underground cities located in the Earth's crust. Two trips to our Hollow Earth in the shuttle craft were on official business between our military and the Inner Earth peoples. The third trip was not on official business, but it was a special trip Billie made to advise the Hollow Earth peoples that it was futile to try to influence our military to become peaceful. At that time, Billie requested permission to stay in the Hollow Earth, but they wouldn't grant permission. They told Billie they had a mission for Billie to carry out on the surface world. That mission is to let outer earth peoples know of the existence of Our Hollow Earth. Also that the Hollow Earth peoples want to be known, and that they are a peaceful people. The more that outer peoples know about the Hollow Earth and the peaceful people that live there, then the more successful they hope they will be in being accepted by outer earthlings when the Hollow Earth peoples do decide to emerge openly to the people of the Earth's outer surface.

Billie says Agharta is a cavern city and that there are two Shambhala's -- one in a cavern city, and another in the Hollow interior. Billie's mission was to interact with the Hollow Earth peoples and report everything learned to superiors in the Air Force. Billie took many pictures and meticulously documented everything seen and heard, and was debriefed completely after each trip.

From what Billie learned, the Hollow Earth people had been interested in trying to convince our military to stop their aggressive behavior as well as their atomic testing which was poisoning the atmosphere on and in the Earth which could harm people in the interior and on the outer surface of the planet. Finally, Billie convinced the Hollow Earth people that it was useless to try to get the military and our government to change their aggressive behavior. It was a waste of time he told them. Billie suggested to the Hollow Earth people that they begin interfacing and contacting the civilian population of the outer Earth instead if they wanted to see a true change on the Earth.

Billie's contacts agreed and said they would start making more civilian contact in the future. They have since told Billie that after the present North Polar Inner Earth expedition, that outer Earth peoples will start to see more contacts in the near future.

Billie says that in other journeys within the tunnel systems they visited many cavern cities and many Inner Earth cities. Billie says that there are tunnels made by the Rand Corporation boring machines, which are not as well made as the Hollow Earth people's tunnels. There are tunnels made by the Hollow Earth people, and tunnels made by cavern cities of other races that live underground, and there are still other ancient tunnels made by the ancient civilizations of Atlantis that was located in the Atlantic Ocean, and Lemuria, which was a Pacific continent called Mu that is now submerged.

Of those tunnels made by surface governments, tunnels join all the capital cities of the world where government leaders can find asylum in case of war or natural disaster. There are many such complexes that exist under all the major cities of the United States, for the same purpose, but which the governments have prepared only for the survival of the government, not the civilian population, in preparation for the close passage of a planet-sized comet that will cause very high winds, earthquakes and tsunamis.

After visiting Telos, the Lemurian city beneath Mt. Shasta, Billie was taken back to Area 51. Later Billie was taken in a tunnel shuttle to the Hollow Earth.

Billie says that the shell of the earth is from 800 to 850 miles thick, and that the center of gravity is about halfway between the outer and inner surfaces of the Earth's shell, and that the inner surface gravity is a little less than one-third the outer surface gravity which allows for the larger stature of the Hollow Earth people, or any surface people that go to the Hollow Earth and stay there for a length of time.

Billie said that the Hollow Earth has an inner sun that gives photosynthesis light that provides life to the Hollow Earth peoples, animals and giant plant life, and that the Hollow Earth country is a most beautiful and harmonious, peaceful place, that even the animals are friendly and able to communicate with humans telepathically and are not aggressive. There are NO meat-eating animals in the Hollow Earth, but all eat vegetation instead. The inner atmosphere, Billie says, is so healthy that no disease can exist there, and if a diseased person coming from the surface would go there, they would be cured just by breathing the air. Before Billie was taken to the Hollow Earth at age 12, Billie had minor childhood sicknesses like colds, and tonsillitis, but when taken to the Hollow Earth, Billie's immune system was fortified to a more healthful state. Since then, Billie's health has deteriorated somewhat due to living on the surface again because of the pollution here but knows that once he returns home to the Hollow Earth, his immune system will return to a completely healthy state.

When Billie arrived at the hollow earth inner surface, they emerged from the shuttle station at the Hollow Earth capitol City of Eden, the main city of the Hollow Earth. It is built around and within the original Garden of Eden on the highest mountain plateau of the inner continent and estimates it is located under the State of Arkansas or close to. Billie says that the world inside our earth has one continent and one ocean, but that there is more land inside the Earth than on the exterior surface.

Billie agrees completely with the Olaf Jansen story, who was Norwegian fishermen that sailed through the North Polar Opening north east of Franz Josef Land, in 1829 -- that the Hollow Earth is exactly as Olaf described in his book, The Smoky God -- because Billie has been there and seen what it is like.

At Eden, Billie was taken before the King of the World, who is also the Great High Priest Over All the Land, to a beautiful pyramid type palace where the King sat on his great marble throne. Billie accompanied by Air Force Colonel McCloud, (and on another subsequent visit with a Colonel Stevenson) were interviewed by the King of the Inner World and asked many questions regarding our outer world, our government and the United States military and what they were up to. Upon returning to Area 51, Billie was completed debriefed and minutely documented all that was learned in Our Hollow Earth.

Billie recounted a time during the military years when he was ordered to fly a US military saucer at Area 51, known as the Sports Craft, the same craft Bob Lazar saw at Area 51. A alien co-pilot instructed Billie on how to fly the craft and accompanied Billie on test flights taken out at night. Billie had been told when assigned to Area 51, that he would not see the light of day while serving there. They flew up over Las Vegas, and other cities and played tag with military jets that were scrabbled to chase their flying saucer and they were able to fly circles around the jets. Billie said the craft was flown by placing the hands on indentations on the control panel that were shaped like hands. Immediately upon placing the hands, Billie had complete control of the craft with just thought commands. If Billie wanted to go in any direction, he just had to think to go in that direction and the craft responded immediately. The craft could make right angle turns at very high speeds, and fly any pattern -- all with no g-force effects. This craft was of our making under the direction of the extraterrestrial, which our military has been building for some time. Billie said they had about 67 saucers built by our military black projects housed at that time at Area 51.

Billie also recounted how the many missing children that have been displaced (as seen on milk cartons) every year throughout the United States are taken to Area 51 where the military black projects are transforming them into programmed biological entities so that they look like hybrid aliens. Their plan is to use the flying saucers they are building and the hybrid entities they are genetically engineering from our children to stage an alien invasion from space to get the whole world to submit to a one world government in defense of the aliens that they have created. When shown this, Billie became so disgusted with the military black projects that he decided not to have anything more to do with this project, and decided to get out of the military.

After Billie's military career was over, Billie was discharged from the Air Force at the Sewart Air Force base, now Smyrna Airport, Tennessee, debriefed at their deprogramming underground facility, and upon orders of superiors, Billie's military files were sealed with NO access by ANYONE. Billie has tried many times to get a record of his military service, but is told those records are sealed, that no-one can see them. Billie was told by military superiors not to speak or talk to anyone of any assignments in the military. However, Billie told them, "I no longer work for you so I will do as I please." For that, Billie's military pension was withdrawn and today lives in Pahrump, Nevada on Social Security disability.

Over the years Billie married and fathered three children who are now grown. The first two children were boys born to the first wife, an Army military policewoman, stationed at Area 51. They were 5 years together. Later that wife went to work for the FBI and so was able to verify Billie's military records. Billie has been married three times, but is now divorced. The second wife Billie married after being discharged from the military. She was a Cherokee Indian, daughter of the Chief and they were married on the Cherokee Reservation. Billie had a daughter by this wife. The last marriage was in Seattle to a UFO MUFON investigator and lasted from 1990-1996.

In August 1986, Billie went to live in Alaska looking for a way to go to the Hollow Earth to go back home. There, Billie enticed several people in an attempt to reach the Hollow Earth by hiring a bush pilot to fly as an expedition team through the north polar opening. Billie arranged through a flight service out of Fairbanks, Alaska to take them in their decommissioned

Navy Albatross seaplane, which is a twin engine seaplane with a boat bottom. It was the same type of seaplane that the Coast Guard uses frequently today -- as seen on the Fantasy Island TV program. Billie requested the pilot to take them to certain coordinates in the Arctic to 87.7 N Lat., 142.2 E Lon that Billie had learned from Admiral Byrd's file at Area 51.

The pilot was concerned about how they would land out there on the ice, but Billie assured him that there would be open Arctic Ocean when they got to those coordinates. The pilot agreed to fly them to those coordinates, land them on the water and drop them off, and that he would be back for them at a certain time in the future three weeks hence. They took some inflatable power boats that they would use to continue their journey from that point on through the polar opening.

Unfortunately, before they took off from Point Barrow, Alaska, one of the expedition members who was a New York Times correspondent, made a phone call to his home office who Billy believes then alerted the military of their flight north.

When they arrived near enough to the polar opening and could see the light beams of the inner sun shining up from the ocean ahead, the pilot was surprised and very afraid and wondered what was going on since they could see the outer sun shining behind them also. Billie assured him that there was nothing to fear, that they were looking at the core of the Earth shining out through a polar opening in the Earth. But before they could drop down to land in the water and depart in their inflatable boats, they were intercepted by two jet fighters from the Alert Air Force Base, on the northern shore of Ellesmere Island, Canada.

The airplane radio crackled and a voice came through, which

stated, "This is Lt. Colonel Travis of the US Air Force Alert Base intercepting team ordering you to turn your aircraft around IMMEDIATELY and be escorted back to Eielson Air Force Base, Alaska, OR YOU WILL BE TERMINATED! You have 5 minutes to comply."

Reluctantly, they started to make their turn around. At the same time, looking through the front view of the aircraft, they suddenly saw three glowing disks appear -- flying saucers -- ahead of them.

The radio crackled again, and another voice came over the radio saying, "Billie, we are here to welcome you to our domain, as you have attempted to enter. We are sorry. You will not make it this time. However, your next journey WILL succeed! Auf Wiedersehen!" And then the three flying saucers suddenly just blinked out.

Rather than disobey orders and get terminated, they decided to turn the aircraft around and do as the US Air force pilot suggested. They retraced their path back to Alaska, where they were instructed to land at Eielson Air Force Base, just southeast of Fairbanks, Alaska. There they were put under bright lights and interrogated and drilled by several agents of the FBI and the National Security Agency. They wanted to make sure they were not terrorists or affiliated with any foreign government. But after they realized they were harmless, they were released and given a stern warning not to tell anyone of what they saw on this trip, and if they were to try that trip again there would be no warning the next time and they would be terminated.

Billie says that many, if not most people in Alaska have gone there with the hopes of going to Our Hollow Earth. Among the interesting persons, Billie met in Alaska was a retired Air Force Col. Jackson of Talkeetna, Alaska that told Billie that in many of his flights into the Arctic out of Eielson Air Force base, near Fairbanks, Alaska, he saw the North Polar Opening and observed many flying saucers going in and coming out of it like bees out of a hive. Billie also tells of another contact he made in Talkeetna who had a ham radio and they tried many times to glance a radio beam off a Hollow Earth satellite that looks like a giant rock that is suspended over the North Polar Opening, down into the Hollow Earth to see if they could make contact with the Hollow Earth peoples that way. Billie says that one evening after his friend had gone to bed that he was able to finally make radio contact with the Hollow Earth people with this ham radio set.

Billie says that when his twin sister, Zuria was taken to an underground think tank around the age of 10, by force to test her abilities, she discovered that they were wanting to dissect her body to see if they could figure out why she had such amazing capabilities and characteristics. She then put out a mental telepathy call to the Hollow Earth for assistance and they came in one of their flying saucers. On a rare occasion that she was allowed to come to the surface, the flying saucer blinked into visibility, and she was beamed up before her captors could grab her--and she was taken home to the Hollow Earth. She is waiting there for Billie to return.

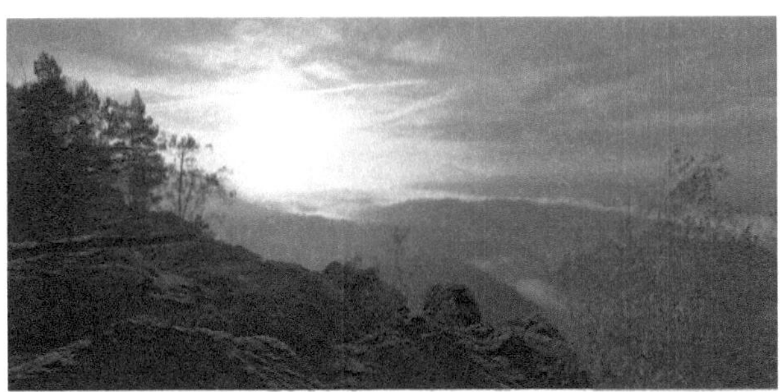

HEALING CRYSTAL WANDS

SANANDA

As always it is wonderful to be with this group, with all of you that join us. We have so much that we're moving toward, all of us are moving toward. So much that is happening but I am not going to get into that area. That I will leave to our dear friend and brother St. Germain. But know that as we continue to move on through this process, this ascension process, this transition that you are all on and that all of us at one time or another have gone through as well in many different and varying ways. And yes even those of you who are going through this process now have also gone through this ascension process if not many times at least once before, so this is not new to your heart's understanding it is only new to your mind. But it is your mind that is creating everything that is happening in your life. It is creating your very existence. But if it is attuned to your heart center then your mind operates from that center and from that high heart center. That is where you are all going. That is what is bringing you up into the higher vibrations, into the higher frequencies and yes, into the higher dimensions. It is your heart mind connection that is doing this.

Those that stay within the mind will remain in the three dimensional experience but those that move into their heart and allow their heart to guide them; allow that small wee whisper from your Higher God Self to guide them, then you will be the ones that will be raising up, soaring into the highest heavens of your being as you continue to move through this process. And then once, when you come to the final moment and you move fully through the ascension and you are fully enmeshed within the fifth dimension and above then you will understand, then you will remember fully who you are and what you have come here to do.

You had a discussion earlier of twin souls. And I share with you now not that it is important to know directly who your twin soul is at this point, (some of you yes, some of you are becoming aware of this,) but understand that it is aspects of yourself. It is aspects of your Higher Self. So there can be many Sanandas, many Yeshuas, many Lady Nadas, many St. Germains, etc. It is not that there is only one. But there is only one twin soul aspect and that is correct. There are many levels though of this aspect. It is not for your mind to understand this at this point. Your three dimensional mind cannot grasp this. Just as your three dimensional mind cannot grasp the idea of a Prime Creator, a Creator Source, but your heart center together with your mind can begin to understand this. And this is where you are all moving toward. This is what this is all about, these gatherings. "Where two or more are gathered in My Name there will I be amongst you." That was said for a reason so that you would understand of the multi-aspects of yourself and how this relates to the reconnection or the re-understanding of that connection with your Higher God Self.

So do not be concerned or consumed with the idea of who you are or who you might've been, but understand that when the moment comes all will be revealed as it needs to be. And as always, you are all in the right place at the right time in the perfect moment. And please just continue to understand that as all of this, all of this continues to unfold right before your eyes.

ST. GERMAIN

As always it is wonderful when I can share some of these moments with you. And these moments are becoming very special, very special indeed. As you continue to move very quickly now toward that understanding, toward that level of oneness that is bringing you to your next highest evolution within yourself and within your selves as a collective.

You all have much to be grateful for, much to be thankful for, because there is only love ahead for you. All of the hate, all of the fear, all of the lower expressions of the lower chakra centers are all being cleared away, cleansed away. The Violet Flame even if you do not use it every day as a visualization although that is helpful even if you do not it is still doing what he needs to across the planet. You are all assisting in this process in any way that you can. And know that there is no greater or lesser part to all of this. You all have a part to play. So believe in yourselves as these things continue to unfold all around you. And it has been in the past and still to some degree this day, for those who have eyes to see and ears to hear these things are opening up more to you. But even to those others now, those ones that are still slumbering; have still not come to an awakening state; even to them, there are changes happening within them. There are spiritual changes happening. Their DNA is being shifted just as yours is. Their third eye centers are beginning to open just as yours is or already has.

There are many understandings that are still yet to come, many indeed. But I ask that you continue to trust, continue to believe in the process because that which we call the Republic — not the New Republic, although it will be new to many. It is really the old Republic. It is the old understanding that is coming forward that is replacing — it is replacing this charade that has been laid across all of you.

It is time to move beyond this charade. It is time to move beyond the falsehoods. It is time to recognize and accept the truth. And as has been said many times, 'the truth shall set you free,' and the truth is there for all to see and all to hear. Just open up. Open up your understandings, open up your heart centers and it will all be revealed to you.

The announcements you have been waiting for are close... very close indeed. We have all been working toward this. For hundreds of years now we have been working toward this moment, this time. For many of you it has been many, many lifetimes you have been working toward this. Now is the time to let go fully and begin to embrace who you truly are. And know that you are so much more than this shell, this body. It is time to understand the true level of your being. It is time to wake up all of you and all of those around you to begin the awakening process.

If you consider your selves already awakened then so be it. But I tell you now you have not even begun yet the awakening. It is going to come upon you when you least expect it. And as it comes upon you it will leave you breathless in many respects. I speak now of the Event, of the Galactic Pulse. When that green light has been given and the Earth receives this grace, this blessing from the high heavens and the Galactic Central Sun the time is short now even from your understanding of time, and my understanding of time when I was there with you.

And that time when the Declaration of Independence was signed I was there to be a part of that expression. I was there to bring this into a level of existence, a level of knowing. I was there just as I am here now. As all that has begun is now coming into fruition. Trust it. Believe it. Do not give up. Do not despair for you are very close now to the beginning of the end and a new beginning; what has been called the beginning of the New Dawn. And that New Dawn is about to break upon all of us.

I AM St. Germain. All of my love, my peace, and the Violet Flame be with each and every one of you. Let it cleanse you. Let it purify you. Let it move through you each and every day so that all that has been, needs be no longer.

Zorra- is a Lemurian, he was present during the time of war between Atlantis and Lemuria. He now lives in Hollow Earth. And because of the high content of copper in Hollow Earth they obtain a turquoise color on their skin. Copper helps them develop super natural abilities. It was Zorra who destroyed the incoming asteroid that was about to hit Russia a few years ago. That extinction level event was recorded by so many people in Russia and I still have that video perhaps someday I will repost it. Zorra prevented the asteroid from hitting the surface of the Earth. When the Disclosure is given either by President Obama or the next president, Zorra will appear as one of the representative of the Lemurian civilization. The president will not only introduce him but also the the Prime Creator, the Galactics such as Sananda and Ashtar. Including the Ascended Masters such as St. Germain. So, when you see the announcement during the Disclosure, these are the people that we will see on our television screen and on the internet.

Adama - is also a Lemurian. But they live in the sub-terranean world which is also connected to Agartha and Hollow Earth. Adama is presently the High Priest of Telos which is a sub-terranean city inside Mt. Shasta.

Zaraya - is also a Lemurian and is the son of Zorra. He was sent to the surface of the Earth to inform the world about the message of Zorra as well as the messages from Prime Creator. Every once in a while, he and his father trade bodies in order to deliver the message. So, instead of just channeling, the swapping of soul and spirit are done so that people are talking and hearing directly from Zorra. Zaraya was also a giant, about 14 feet tall. Before they sent him they needed to shrink his height into the size of a toddler, they put him on a chamber and gradually he started to shrink and they deposited him and his sister in Texas. They also alter his DNA to better match to what we have on Earth surface. And then he was adopted by the Woodards family in 1961 and they gave him the name as Billie Faye Woodard. When he grew up his memory started coming back. And his father Zorra- appeared to him to help him remember who he is and what his mission was.

The Lemurians are the pioneer settlers who responded to the call of inhabiting the surface of a planet. And this was something that has never been done before in any part of the Universe. Because all the planets in the universe are all hollow inside, meaning all their civilizations are residing inside the interior of every planet. And so every planet has a northern and southern polar entry points which acts as a gateway. The spherical dome interior of a planet is ideal and optimal design by the Creator for every being to live into. Not only the inhabitants are protected from the harsh elements present on the surface of the planet such as various storms, earthquakes, meteor showers but also from invasion from another planet that are rogue, not part of the Galactic Federation.

The Lemurians came from planet Lemur and the ancestors of the Lemurians came from the Sirius star system. They arrived on planet called Earth which is also called as Terra and having a Galactic name as Gaia. They occupied a very large areas of the Earth, from the regions of western Russia and all the way to the Pacific. At the time, it was not yet called Pacific but instead it was simply called as MU which was a nickname for Lemuria. The Pacific was not yet covered by ocean water; it was just a vast land that will be converted into a paradise on Earth.

In order to make the Earth habitable by various kinds of animals, they made the basin of the Pacific to have a number of terrains. They sculpted the terrains making the western part of the Pacific deeper than any other areas of the Pacific. And when the formations of terrains was done then they were able to bring with them the Dinosaurs and Mammoths from planet Lemur and this include the teradactyl - the flying dinosaur.

By now you can imagine the size of these animals. The sheer size of a dozen or so of these creatures cannot possibly fit inside the biggest oil tanker of the world today. They brought several of them on the land of Lemuria this includes the so called T-Rex. All the Dinosaurs and Mammoths are all vegetarian. They are not aggressive or violent type of creatures. You can actually take a ride with these animals and they will let you into their backs as though you are riding a horse or an elephant. You can do the same thing with the Teradactyl as they can let you fly with them and soar the highs and lows of the terrains of Mu. The teeth and the claw of these animals are just for the shredding the barks of a tree. They are not carnivorous and they will never eat any other animals or humans.

The last two decades or so we saw the discoveries of various dinosaurs and mammoths found on the Siberian region which is also part of Lemuria. The dinosaurs and mammoths surprisingly they discovered when dissected to open their stomach they found that the contents of their stomachs are just plant based diet. There was no meat whatsoever. And this was consistent to all the dinosaurs that were found frozen in the ice of Siberia and this includes the mammoths.

If we remove all the water of the Pacific Ocean (just for illustration purposes) you will see that it was sculpted for the very purpose of accommodating large species of animals. And if there is no water that covers the Pacific you can find some entryways or caves that was converted into caverns for the Lemurians to live into. One of these entryways was discovered recently just off the coast of southern California. Underneath the water of the beach when following the contours of the terrain you will find such entry ways like a big cave which leads you to subterranean location. The Lemurians also built viewing stations. One example is the one submerge underwater on the southern islands of Japan called Yonoguni. This island is near Taiwan and northern Philippines. If you search diligently this island including the underwater areas you can still find the remnants of the Lemurian civilization. But because its been a long time, some of those relics are already severely damaged from water erosion. The viewing platform was designed in order for people to see the panoramic view of the paradise called Mu as it gives you the wide angle view of the surroundings as well as the deeper terrains where the giant animals are located. This is also a good starting point if you want to ride the flying teradactyl as you can enjoy the thrill of it diving into the deeper terrain from the top of the mountain. All the islands of the Pacific these includes the Hawaiian islands, micronesia, Easter Islands, New Zealand, Fiji, Nauru, Guam, Saipan, Japan, Philippines and etc. are all the upper portions of the mountains of Lemuria. And each of these mountains have a network subterranean residential living spaces that has been kept secret for thousands of years! And they are all interconnected.

This means you can ride an underground tunnel using a shuttle that has no wheels but is magnetically levitated on all areas of the tunnel to secure safety and it travels faster than the latest maglev trains built on the surface of the world by either Japan, China and Korea. With this mode of underground transport, you can reach Easter island in a matter of 30 minutes. You can ride these high speed underground shuttle and you can reach either Japan, the Philippines, Australia and even Tibet in 30 minutes. By the way, do you know why some of the scriptures during First Century AD was able to survive all these thousands of years, including the Gospel written by Mary Magdalene? It was all possible because of the existence of this extensive line of network of underground passageways that connects most of the Lemurian regions. Because of this mode of underground transport they were able to move not just passengers but also cargoes of all kinds.

Some of the original first century writings of Mary Magdalene was preserved by the use of these underground passageways with high speed levitating shuttles; and was able to avoid confiscation by the Romans. The Roman Emperor Constantine confiscated much of the first century scriptures and burned them. And after that they edited the Bible. That is why the oldest Bible in the Vatican only dates back to the third century AD.

And today it is called as the Agarthan network. Which not only comprise the underground passageways but also the cities underneath those cities. Yes they built cities underneath those Lemurian mountains which is connected to a more underground residential living. There is an ancient underground city underneath the base of Mt. Fuji in Japan and the same thing with the mountains in northern Philippines and of course Mt. Shasta in California and they are all interconnected via underground tunnels. You can take a ride in any of this underground shuttles and it will take you quickly to any destination you wish. The difference with the technology of the Lemurians with what we have today in the surface of the world is that their knowledge and technology is more advance than ours. For example, when you are riding any of their underground shuttles you cannot feel any of the G-force or inertia. Even though you are traveling in the speed of sound their technology can cancel the inertia of its forward motion as though you are just inside a non-moving stationary room. And this kind of technology can also be seen with their aeroships that fly inside the Hollow Earth and sometimes we see them on the surface of the world and we call them UFOs. This means you can even drink a cup of coffee or tea inside the shuttle or their aeroship even though its moving extremely fast and it will not suffer any spill of that liquid as the containment inside the ship and the shuttle are not subjected by the Earth's gravitational pull.

Along with the animals they also brought with them the plants and trees and they populated the Lemurian regions with so much vegetations that really was called the Paradise of Earth. Mu was indeed called paradise and heaven on earth. But the Garden of Eden is not found inside the regions of Lemuria and neither in any other surface areas of the Earth. This is because, the garden of Eden is located INSIDE the Hollow Earth. Let me draw the distinctions. The solid crust of the Earth is only 800 miles in thickness and this is where the subterranean region is located. And after the 800 miles is an open interior Hollow Space called Hollow Earth. The Garden of Eden is inside the Hollow Earth. There is a city inside the Earth called Eden and that is the original location of the garden mentioned in the bible.

During and after the war between Atlantis and Lemuria that was the time that the Lemurians started moving into the Hollow Earth. The Lemurians or what we call the people of ancient Lemuria transferred and or migrated to these two regions: a) Subterranean crust of the Earth b) The Hollow Interior of the Earth which was originally inhabited by the Aryanis.

How do they look like?

The Lemurians are very tall they range from 13 to 18 feet tall. For example Zorra from Hollow Earth is also a Lemurian, he is 15 feet tall. His wife Sarriya is around 13 to 14 feet tall. While those in the subterranean region on the crust of the Earth their height is around 8 to 11 feet tall. The Lemurians in terms of race are a combination of caucasian looking people as well as oriental (asian) and some are similar to the Pacific islanders.

Their skin colors varies from Blue, Turquiose (mix green & blue), white and etc. While their hair color ranges from golden yellow, orange, red, black, and blonde. This is the reason why when you go visit India you will find their gods (not Gods) are beings with blue skin. This is because these blue skinned or turquoise colored people came from inside the Earth and they are part of the Lemurian civilizations. Another example in the Phillipines there is a folklore or stories of giants who came out of the mountains and they usually come out when its already near sunset.

The remains of some of the Lemurians who were victims of the war between Atlantis and Lemuria can be found underneath Tibetan mountains near China and also the deserts of Gobi. When they excavated these regions they saw humans that are very tall and have red and blonde hairs. And these are not Europeans. The same thing with the pyramids of China, inside you can see the mummified remains of Lemurian people and most of them have a caucasian features having red hair and etc.

What does these mean?

This means that the human body regardless of race is only a temporary dwelling place. It can be discarded, it can be replaced with a new one. You can either choose any of the default designs of various races as what race you choose to have as a physical body is not very important. Because the physical body is no different from a garment that we wear. Our clothes in our closet have varying different kinds of colors and different kinds of styles, designs and patterns. It works the same way with the physical body. The assortment of choices of different races are just a matter of design and its DNA. In other words, we are not the body that we currently have. Just as you can choose various brands of cars whether Ford, GMC, Toyota, Jeep, Nissan, Saab, BMW, Maserati, Lamborghini, Renault, Kia and so on. The same thing with the human body the Lemurians can choose the type of body they can have. Remember, you are the driver of the vehicle and you are not the car, instead you are the one who is driving the car. The car is not you. And this analogy is very applicable to the human body. We are not our body. The body is not you. You are the person inside the body. And you are the one who is operating your own body telling it where to go and what to do, just like you would with a car.

The Lemurians are also capable of transforming and or morphing into another body either human or animal and its usually a body of an animal such as birds, eagles and some four footed animals. They are also capable of dematerializing that allows them to pass through walls regardless of the thickness of it. For example, if you record the lenticular clouds that comes out of Mt. Shasta and or Mt. Fuji, you can see that it originated inside the mountain. They applied the technology of dematerializing their spacecraft into lenticular clouds. And when you follow this clouds you will find that eventually it will dissipate and disappear as vapor into the sky as they are already on their way going offworld. The Lemurians themselves already admitted that those lenticular clouds are camouflaged spacecrafts.

For now, we find these capabilities of the Lemurians are out of touch with our present reality and technology. Because it does sounds like a science fiction. But it is not. This is because we on the surface of the planet are subjected to a very limited lifespan by incarnating allover again and again repeatedly to several lifetimes on different human bodies. And by going through those process we lose the memories of the past. In addition to that the secret rulers of this world are constantly stealing and hiding the already acquired knowledge and technologies for their own advantage. We all know that they suppressed the discoveries and inventions of Tesla. Did you know that for more than a hundred years now that there are scores of inventions from around the world that have been confiscated and was hidden underneath the basement of the US government building? This was revealed by the people of Hollow Earth. And so we have to discover all over again what we already knew before in previous lifetimes. And this is the main reason why you find yourself interested in some activities or studies that you feel you resonated with it is because in your previous lifetimes you were once engaging in those activities. Now, this is not the case for the Lemurians as they never grow old and never die as their technologies are designed for optimal living that can prolonged peoples lifespan to several thousands of years. While we on the surface constantly forget what we already know in previous lifetime and then have to be reborn into another body only to re-learn what we already knew before. And this cause us so much time delay with our knowledge of science and technologies. But say for example if you have a time budget of at least three thousand years of mastering the tricks of playing tennis or any other sports, then you can defeat any grand slam champion out there. By having sufficient and enough time to practise some crafts, activities, sciences, martial arts or sports then you can eventually refine and further improve to perfection anything that you put your heart and mind into accomplishing. With Lemurians this is something that they have for eons of time as they really have ETERNITY to improve and study things. This means they have the technology that they already mastered and perfected for eons and eons of time while we are just barely scratching the surface of those technologies and or scientific knowledge.

Another example is the art and science of holographic image combined with the technology of force field. Do you know why the North Pole and South Pole appears to be sometimes Hollow with open space and then sometimes it just plainly covered with ICE? The answer is the holographic projections technology. They can project an image onto it making it look like it is covered with ice glacier, but in truth, it is actually open like a hole of the donut (see the illustrations). In addition to the Holographic image, they also combined it with a force field. And so when you bump into it you feel like it is solid. But when they turn off the force field, then you can pass through the polar opening and be able to get inside the Hollow Earth. This is exactly what happened with Admiral Byrd who flew to the North and South Pole and the Agarthans turned off the holographic image of ice and he was able to see inside the Hollow Earth, where the trees are bigger than the biggest trees we have on the surface of the Earth. By turning off the force field, Admiral Byrds airplane was able to go inside the Hollow Earth and saw the small interior central sun inside the Earth.

Now, the question is how do we meet the Lemurians and learn from them?

The Lemurians are good people. We can either visit them or we wait for them to come out and congratulate us for the celebration is at hand for the New Golden Age of the Earth. They will do this when the Disclosure are given by the worlds government about the benevolent presence of the Galactics and the people of Hollow Earth including the Lemurians. They were hoping president Obama will do the disclosure in his remaining final days in office. But because of the complications with the Clintons controversy it might not happen with Obama.

But there is still some chance that he will have the guts to tell the truth about the reality of extra terrestrial presence as well as the Lemurian people of Agarthan network inside the Earth. And if President Obama will not be able to announce disclosure. Then, the responsibility of disclosure may be turned over to the next president.

The difficulties with Obama is that since he is only a CEO of a private corporation which is the USA corp. then it means he have higher ups that he needs to answer to. And that prevents him from doing completely what he wanted to do. The Lemurians know that Obama is a good person and that he is a light-worker but because of his limitations that is doing significant constraints preventing him from doing the right thing and therefore things like disclosure and stopping wars in the middle east can be very challenging for him as the secret society that is giving him orders of what to say and do are really not good people, they are very evil. And he have to obey them. And that is the main problem with President Obama, but deep inside Obama is a good and genuine person and the Galactics knows this.

The original initial plan was that there will be a Disclosure that will be done by Obama announcing it lives on television and along with him are the members of the Galactic Federation, Ashtar, Sananda, St. Germain, Prime Creator and Zorra from Hollow Earth. But if President Obama will announce it then he has to do it between now and November 8 as his term of office will end in the coming days. Will it make any difference if he decided to do it after the said November 8, 2016? Although, it will be more convincing if it happens while he is still in office, but when his term of office ends, then maybe the ideal thing to do is that to do an announcement when he is already free from the responsibility that binds him from the US corporation. That means, he does not have to obey them. Then he will be free to say what he needs to be said and announce what should be announced in the first place. He may also opt to include the incoming interim president of the US, perhaps Paul Ryan? to make the joint announcement of the Disclosure that has been long overdue since the days the Galactics met with President Eisenhower and Kennedy (JFK). When the Agarthans and Lemurians will come out to meet us people on the surface of the world, it will mean that the cabal has been defeated and there will be a global celebration as earlier outlined a few years before by St. Germain, Zorra and the Galactic Federation.

The New World is coming, a world where people will no longer be under the influence and control of the bad secret rulers of this world. And when that happens the Lemurians will come out and meet with us. And they call it the "Emergence". It will fulfill what Ashtar said prophetically that Lemuria the paradise and heaven on Earth will come back. It will also fulfill the prophecy of the book of Revelation saying: "And there was a new Earth, and there was no more sea." Yes, that means they will bring back Lemuria to the way it was in the beginning. They will transport the whales and some other kinds of fish and bring them back to Sirius and Pleaides. And then they will reduce the worlds ocean and what will be left are just a number of rivers and lakes. This maybe one of the primary reason why the delegation from Sirius brought a mothership in which according to Zorra is twice the size of the Earth. I still have a copy of this footage of the mothership from Sirius that is twice the size of the Earth. Definitely it can accommodate the worlds ocean water and bring back the lands of Lemuria.

ST. MICHAEL THE ARCHANGEL

Some years ago, when I was a young seminarian, I served with an Episcopal priest who greatly disappointed me in conversation one day by telling me that he saw "no need" for angels. "There's nothing that angels are described as doing that the Holy Spirit could not do instead." This kind of heavenly economy had never been offered to me as a theological reason before. When I thought about it, I realized that there was nothing that we could do that the Holy Spirit couldn't do better, and wondered whether we existed. It seemed silly to me to posit something as not existing simply because you saw no need for it.

Later that week I was in a prayer group with this same priest (in his parish where I worked). It was a fairly informal group, and I have to confess to pure naughtiness when I said to the group, "Father said he sees no need for angels." I don't know what I expected, but the response was a sudden torrent of people sharing stories about angels that were purely wonderful. It included a story by an elderly woman who told of seeing an angel by the bed of her dying child. By the end of the evening, my priest friend had recanted and professed a belief in angels.

That is a story from the confusing time of an Anglican seminarian. What do you do when your professor and mentor just ups and denies a cardinal doctrine of the faith? I didn't know at the time, so I probably did something wrong – though the outcome was good.

In the years since then I have had occasion in sermon or in a class to share a story about an encounter with an angel, or the intervention and help of an angel (I have a few such stories to tell). Without fail the result has been the same as that first night in a prayer group in Chicago. The story I tell is met with a torrent of similar stories. It seems that many people have angelic encounters but (at least in the circles I was in) were afraid to tell anybody.

Apparently, if you live in a two-storey universe and you tell about an encounter with a second-floor creature, some people are afraid of the consequences. Thus we have the strange phenomenon of living in a one-story universe where God is everywhere present, where the holy angels surround us moment by moment, and at the same time, we have a great conspiracy of silence not to tell anyone about how things really are. Secularism is just one large myth.

Tonight my wife and I prayed the Akathist to the Archangel Michael (we were offering intercession for a friend). At the end of the prayers my wife said quietly to me, "St. Michael has always been a good friend to us." It was a time for me to pause and remember how many times through 33 years of marriage we have stood together and asked St. Michael to come to our aid. Sometimes it has been through our own need, other times for the needs of others. But what we have known has been the faithfulness of the "Chief Captain of the Heavenly Hosts" to do battle for us and protect us in all of our spiritual battles.

Who Are the Seven Archeiai? You are probably familiar with the archangels yet not with the archeia. An archeia is the feminine complement of an archangel and thus wields tremendous energies of the Spirit in her service to mankind often in a gentler and somewhat more feminine manner than her masculine counterpart. Since we know the names of the archeiai of the Seven Archangels, we may call to each of them to bless us with their particular aspect of God's consciousness for the color ray upon which they serve. Each of the Seven Archeiai: Faith, Christine, Charity, Hope, Mary, Aurora and Amethyst is a powerful intercessor for mankind, answering the prayers of those in distress in very specific and, at times, mysterious ways.

The Rosary—A Prayer for All Time

Disciples of the Spirit who have offered rosaries and prayers to the Blessed Mother may be aware that there is a long tradition of various types of rosaries that have been given over the years since Jesus' life on earth. The original rosary given centuries ago looked much different than that which is given within the Catholic Church of today. Rather than a single prayer for all time, the rosary has become an evolution of devotion. Over the years, various mystics and saints, in communion with Jesus and other heavenly beings, have added to the hallowed tradition of the rosary. The Rosary of Faithis another step in this divine evolutionary process known as progressive revelation.

A Garland of Roses

Each rosary is, in reality, a spiritual garland of roses created by giving various prayers, most often including the "Hail Mary" which honors the words of the Archangel Gabriel spoken to Mary when she was a temple virgin, spending much of her time in prayer and meditation upon the heaven world. This rosary continues the tradition of pouring forth devotion to the Blessed Mother Mary, Queen of the Angels, who has been so instrumental in answering the prayers of the faithful over the centuries.

A Rosary for the Anchoring of God-Government

This Rosary of Faith is the fulfillment of a request made to David Lewis by the Ascended Masters El Morya and Lanello. When the program for a weekend conference in Washington, D.C. in late January 2007 was given, David was also asked to have ready a completed version of a new Rosary of Faith, wherein participants would invoke the light of all seven complements of the archangels, primarily the Archeia Faith, the consort of beloved Archangel Michael. Since Washington, D.C. is the blue-ray focus and throat chakra for the United States of America, it seemed fitting that faith should be concentrate through a new type of rosary for the protection of our nation's government and its leaders. Those of all nations may give this new rosary for the anchoring of God-government in their own country and in all nations, maximizing the light of these prayers on behalf of all peoples.

Faith Is the First and Essential Virtue After which All Others Follow

In all spiritual traditions unless there be faith and belief, the light of wisdom's fires and the fulfillment of love in all things does not ensue. Works alone do not allow us entrée into the kingdom of God but inspired works of compassion born of spiritual knowledge and faith flow from a profound oneness of Spirit.

Create a Cosmic Corona of Blessing Around Yourself

By invoking the light of all seven arches in this rosary, we create a rainbow radiance, a cosmic carona of God's tender blessing around us. Our halos shine not only with the emerald color of Mary's presence but with the specific pastel glory of each of this angelic mothers who can nurture us in many sublime ways. Thus, no matter what day of the week we choose to give this rosary, we can have access to all of the "seven sisters" whose manifestation of light complement each other in ways great and small.

Invoke the Presence of the Angelic Choirs to Expand Your Consciousness

We know that singing our prayers opens our hearts in a profound way, and we've been told that hymns of praise invoke the presence of the angelic choirs. In this rosary we pray to the nine choirs of angels, each of these focusing a specific aspect of

God's radiance at a different level of vibration in the heaven world. Some choirs live and move and have their being closer to the Godhead while others work more closely with mankind. By attuning to each choir's specific purpose and work, we can more readily expand our own consciousness to the level of these angelic beings. And thereby they, too, may work more closely with us.

Commune with the Angels and Enter Cosmic Grace

Many of us who have dedicated our lives to the service of mankind are actually embodied angels, and thus we easily resonate with these beautiful presences that are often so close at hand to us though we often know it not. By cosmic law they cannot act within our dimension unless we invoke them by intention. Now you have in this rosary a means of communing with these wonderful friends of light and entering into their world of cosmic grace in a simple, new way.

ONE WHO SERVES

Greetings to you!

I am coming in very loud and clear because there is some here that is snoring. [Laughter] (must not have come back from the meditation) We need to wake up! That was St. Germain did he not say wakeup? Well here in the room wakeup people. It is time, it is certainly time not only to wake up, not only to become aware of who you are but to move on in expression, move on to these higher vibrations that are so close to coming upon you. You each one are beginning to experience this. We hear this earlier in your tales of your animals and birds and all of these things. And all of this is happening for reason and it is happening as part of this process as you are moving into these higher vibrations. But understand they are not moving down into the lower vibrations with you, you are moving up into the higher vibrations with them. As you move up into the higher vibrations the birds the cats the dogs the tigers, all of this will be a part of the expression with you, that love expression. That is where you are headed each and every one of you. And as Archangel Michael said two weeks ago as we are finding it as he said, 'be ready for experiences that you are going to have in your dreams and your waking state and your visions.' All of this is coming. All of this is going to be part of your expression as this veil continues to drop. Moment by moment inch by inch this veil is dropping and pretty soon people it is going to be gone. And do you know what it is going to be like for you when it is gone? Do you have any idea what that is going to be like? No you do not have an idea yet because it is beyond your wildest imagination of what that will be like. It will be as if a cloud, a cloud that has been over you for your entire existence is suddenly lifted and the light comes shining through that wasn't coming through before. Can you visualize this? Can you understand what we are saying here? It is going to be grand and brilliant beyond your imaginations, but before that can happen you must continue to go about your daily life as you do but each and every day as you move through the moments of your day, find that joy in every moment. Find that expression of love in every moment. Move yourselves into the higher vibration in every moment that you can. Every moment that you can, especially when you are outside in nature see the beauty of nature. It is all around you. This is what these words, these hummingbirds, these various animals are trying to bring to you to tell you that it is a new day, it is a new dawn. Begin to understand that and let it express through you. Okay?

We get off our soapbox now [laughter] and are ready for questions. And no I am not the one who is the, what you would call, the standup comedian but I can also at times bring a little fun and enjoyment and cheer and get you laughing and all of this. But that is because I have been taking lessons from the other one. And as you heard earlier at one time or another he has been taking lessons from none other than Robin Williams. Yes! Believe it or not he is here with us in many respects and he has been giving us quite a run for our money I must tell you. So I guess I might be considered One Who Serves number four. Okay? Just in case, you were wondering.

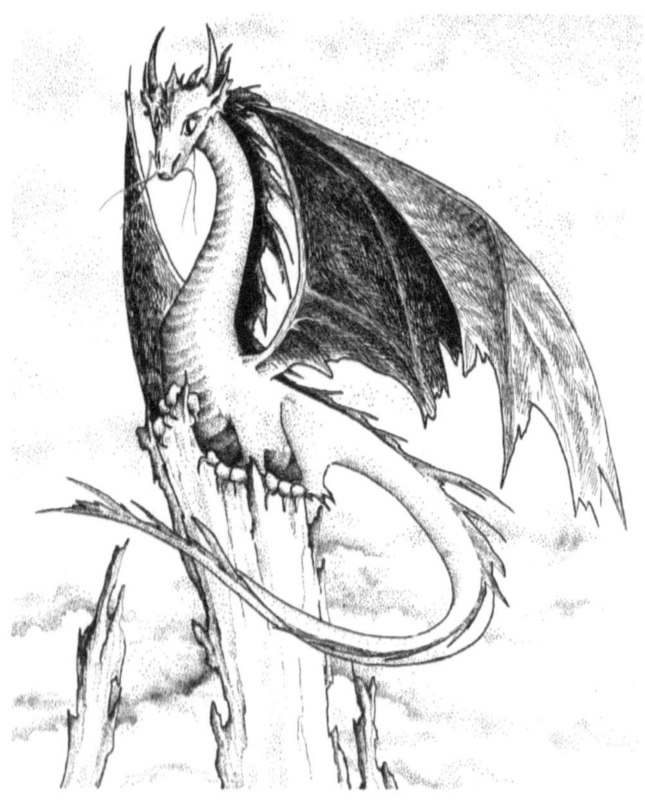

MESSAGES FROM THE HOLLOW EARTH

Explanation of our Hollow Earth

Not just our Earth, but all planets are Hollow! Planets are formed by hot gases thrown from a sun into an orbit, and the shell of planets is created by gravity and centrifugal forces and the POLES REMAIN OPEN and lead to a hollow interior. This process forms a Hollow Sphere with an Inner Sun, smoky in color, which gives off soft and pleasant, full spectrum sunlight, making the inside surface highly conducive to growth of vegetation and human life... with only a long-long day and no nights.

The Hollow Earth beings are very spiritually evolved and technologically advanced, and live inside the interior core of our Hollow Earth. These advanced civilizations live in peace and brotherhood in the Center of our Earth, which contains an Inner Central Sun, with oceans and mountains still in their pristine state.

The Hollow Earth cavity is still in its pristine state because they don't walk or build upon their land. There are no buildings, shopping malls or highways. They travel in electromagnetic vehicles that levitate a few inches above ground. They walk along streams, rivers, and oceans and climb mountains - but that's the extent of their foot contact with the ground. They leave the rest of their land to nature, because it's nature's land too.

The governing city within the Hollow Earth is called Shamballa. It is located inside the very center of the planet and can be accessed through the holes at either the North or South poles. The Northern and Southern Lights that we see in our skies are actually reflections from our Hollow Earth's Inner Central Sun, which emanates from her Hollow Core.

They use free energy to light up their cities, homes, and tunnels. They use crystals, coupled with electromagnetism, which generates a small sun with full-spectrum lighting that lasts for half a million years, and gives them all the power they need.

The Earth's crust is approximately 800 miles from the outer to the irmer surface. Because our Earth is Hollow, and not a solid sphere, the center of gravity is not in the center of the Earth, but in the center of its crust, which is 400 miles below the surface.

The source of Earth's magnetic field has been a mystery. The Inner Sun at the center of Earth is the mysterious power source behind the Earth's magnetic field.

There are entry caverns all over the Earth, where interactions can take place. Only some are currently open. Nikola Tesla, the genius inventor of electrical technology, is now living inside the Hollow Earth. He began to receive information in the latter part of the 1800' s and discovered that: "electric power is everywhere present in unlimited quantities and can drive the world's machinery without the need of coal, oil, gas or any other of the common fuels." In the 1930's the tunnels entrances and passageways were closed off by the Hollow Earth civilizations because 'corporations' at that time were misusing Tesla's technology to gain entrance into the Inner Earth. The Hollow Earth's two main portals are at the Holes at the Poles, which were closed off in the year 2000 because our governments were setting detonations at the Poles to blow open entrances into their world. They have installed a magnetic force field around Earth's polar openings to further camouflage the entrances. This way, the openings are protected from air and land sightings. In the past there were entrances to the Library of Porthologos on the surface. One such entrance was the Library of Alexandria, which was destroyed by fire in A.D. 642.

There is more landmass inside (3/4 land and 1/4 water) and the land is more condensed than ours. Everything in the Hollow Earth is very carefully maintained to balance the ecological system of all life forms that reside there.

There are several million Catharians currently residing in the Hollow Earth. There are Catharians who have incarnated as humans on the surface. There are also Catharians that live on the planet Jupiter. The tallest Catharian is 23 feet tall. There are 36,000 humans from our surface who now live inside the Earth. Over the last 200 years approximately 50 surface humans went inside to live. Over the last 20 years only 8 went inside to live.

Introduction from Adama

We have traveled extensively together, attended more council meetings together than you can count, and have spent time together in each other's homes and cities. work intimately and his entourage in Catharia, and we spend much of our time, when we are visiting the Hollow Earth, in the great Library of Porthologos, where we continue our learning in the vastness of its portals.

We want you to know that our connection to each other is as one link on a fence. We in Telos work as one with our brothers and sisters in Catharia, as our mission is to bring the Earth and surface humanity into her ascension. Although our civilizations are based on the same Divine Laws of Creation, our experiences as a culture differ, due to our different geographical locations on Earth. But this is our only difference, and makes our interactions more fruitful as we each bring different riches to the table of our council meetings.

Mikos has been a close friend and companion traveler of mine for eons of Earth time, and we work together closely to join all the civilizations on and in Earth together into one United Earth World Colony, so that our planet will be readied to make the great trip with the rest of our Milky Way Galaxy into a higher state of evolution. Our location in our new position in the Milky Way Galaxy has been prepared and is waiting for for us all to return home to.

As you read the pages in this book, your heart will be prepared to make the journey with us into our new home of Light everlasting. We beckon you to travel with us through these pages of great insight and delight, and learn the true history of your planet Earth, and how other civilizations live embedded beneath your surface and below your periphery of vision.

Our book is a prerequisite to this sequel, in terms of establishing our Telosian history and lifestyle as contrasted to that of the Hollow Earth inhabitants, who are only a step below us. We are all ONE and the same, and yet different in myriad ways; just as your nations and people are on the surface. Both of our civilizations chose to live underground in isolation from the surface population, so we could evolve in tranquility and peace.

So ride with us in your thoughts, and travel to the innermost depths of our Earth, and you will find the lost Garden of Eden your bible talks about. It is right here, in the center of your Earth, waiting to be explored by you, the reader. We welcome you in. I am Adama.

Welcome

Welcome! Welcome to the beginning of a marvelous, and for many a seemingly unbelievable journey. My name is Mikos, and you are about to enter through these pages a realm that pre dates history as you know it. A realm of fancy and fantasy, a realm of surrealistic beauty and eternal changelessness; a place that has been hidden to all but a few souls who have ventured here in the past by invitation only.

For some, this journey presented revelations beyond time. For all, it changed the course of their understanding in the world in which they lived, and ultimately their entire lives. In reading the humble messages of these pages which lie before you, you are about to meet one of those people, Dianne Robbins . . . a beautiful, gracious, and the gentlest of souls, whose life is intimately connected and bound together with the Cetacean life which reside beneath the waters of your world.

What you are about to read is no less a miracle, one which many years from now will bear the finest and richest of fruits. The fruit of knowledge...the fruit of gentle wisdom... the fruit of truth, unity, compassion, and endless joy and love... by which life was always meant to flourish.

Please accept this invitation now and begin a journey into the mysterious world in which I live. Welcome to the Hollow Earth. My people welcome you with Joy, Love, and Peacefulness. May all your journeys in literature be as wondrous and beautiful as the information that lies before you now.

Welcome, dearest children. Welcome to the Library of Porthologos, where the history of all dimensions are shared, stored, and preserved. Where nothing is lost and where every life that has ever existed has been woven into the meaning in the tapestry. Our world is one in which no item as small, or as seemingly insignificant, has been overlooked. This is a Library. A Library nestled beneath the long, deep silence of the Aegean Sea. We, who live and work here, welcome you.

Welcome to the world that awaits your discovery, not only in literature, in written text, but also in form, where through us and a limitless supply of imagination can bring to life the greatest minds that have ever existed. Nothing is lost here.

You can meet and interact with all of creation when you enter through our doors.

You are about to enter a Library...

The Lost City...

The Library of Alexandria!

You Have Waited Thousands of Years to Hear Our Messages.

Greetings from the Hollow Earth! I am Mikos and I dwell inside your Earth. I am reaching up to you in consciousness, to impart our frequency to you as you read the words on these pages of our book. These pages are sacred, for its content contains the mighty power to change the world - if but enough surface folk read them. This is our purpose for dictating our messages to you. It is to hasten change on the surface so that people will once again be connected to their divine self and source of inner guidance.

You have waited for thousands of years to hear our messages, and it is only now that the vibration is high enough for us to come forward and speak to you. These messages you read, come directly through our hearts, relayed from the heart of God. Your heart is God's receptacle - so open it wide, my dear readers, and receive our words directly into your heart - where their vibrations will raise your consciousness enough to meld into us directly as your eyes perceive our words.

We await the great day when we will be able to show our selves to you, when you will be able to peer directly into our eyes and fathom the God within our souls - including yours. Many are now still separated from the Lord God I AM of their being, but our purpose for these messages is to bring you the reality of your own God Selves and help you connect to the Light within your own soul.

Life is about connecting - not disconnecting into separate units, as your density and negativity and limitation on the surface caused you to do. Life is a flow of energy, connecting everyone, everywhere, simultaneously. We invite you to be in this flow, and flow with our thoughts and our heartbeat as you read our words carried to the surface on the winds of telepathy - winds that bring our thoughts and feelings into your heart space - for you to also access as you learn to resonate with our vibration. As you think of Us, you will feel a heightened sense of being as our energy cascades into you. It is a physical sensation that is unmistakable. Move into it - for it is Us - making contact with you - consciousness contact - and it feels like energy currents flowing through you, currents of heightened sensitivity and divine bliss, putting you into a protected space of peace during our connection, that lingers about you for the remaining day. We offer you this, as a gift freely given as you read our words. We've been calling to you for so long, and now through this book to the world, you are hearing us. We are joyously anticipating your heart contact and are ready and eager to respond to your thoughts. So time into us, sit quietly, and feel our vibration engulf your physical body and raise your energy field. We wait for your call.

The Library of Porthologos

Our Library Holds the Records of the Universe.

Greetings from the Center of the Earth! My name is Mikos, and I am a resident of the city of Catharia. I am talking to you from the Library of Porthologos, located in the Hollow Earth beneath the Aegean Sea.

I am very old by definition. I span eons of time in the same body. I have been able to compile Earth's records in the Library of Porthologos, where all Earth's history has been preserved. Our library is immense and extensive and holds the records of the Universe not just Earth. We can study the history of all planets and solar systems and learn everything about life everywhere. Such is our library's capacity. Not only can we read about it, but we can experience it all firsthand from our crystals that store the memories of all events. So we can access these events, learn from them, and solve our problems easily and with the best possible outcomes for all involved.

Our Library Guides the Evolution of a Planet

I am a librarian and researcher by trade, but a statesman (although we have no states) and ambassador for the whole Earth. 1 venture out on journeys to other star systems and galaxies and arrange for their records to be transferred to our library here in Porthologos for safekeeping. We house all the records in our Universe so that someday all people, everywhere in our Universe, will be able to come here to peruse their records and learn their wisdom to avert the negative and ensure the positive outcome of all events. This is the purpose of a library - it is to give guidance for the evolution of a society and a planet so that the people can live and evolve in peace and prosperity - not negativity and war.

All conceivable situations and answers are found in our library, ready to be assimilated by you. As soon as peace prevails on the surface, we can open our library doors to you and accompany you inside. We long for this day, which is assuredly dawning. As we draw closer to our glorious reunion, we send you our everlasting love from below and hope you will return it on your out-breath, where we can set up a circle of love revolving around and through our beloved Earth. I am Mikos, love incarnate.

Our Galactic Connection

The Story of the Hollow Earth Inhabitants

Greetings from the Center of the Earth, an inhabitant below the Earth's surface, enfolded in the Hollow globe deep on the inside space of Earth, as lifeforms circle around and above us on the surface. You are on the rim, so to speak, while we dwell in the cradle, which is safe and secure from outside forces of chaos that are currently raging around you.

As many of you are now familiar with Telos, but not really familiar with the Hollow Earth inhabitants, we would like you to hear our story now. We are a very advanced race of Beings who have never resided on the surface. We have come from other planets in your solar system and other galaxies from the far out reaches of space. We came here to oversee the Earth, and we came here to continue our own evolution without interference from any race or ET's. We are securely encased in the core of the Earth, sufficiently to protect us from all outside intrusion, so that we can evolve as quickly as we can in order to secure this planet as an outpost of Love and Light. For the quicker we can evolve, the quicker we can come to the surface to help struggling humanity gain its freedom into the Light of God's Love. This is why you have not seen or heard from us. It is because we have self-imposed this seclusion.

We now wish you to acknowledge Us, standing free in the Light of God, in the midst of you; constantly radiating out our Light and Love to you to grasp and hold onto as we pull you closer and closer to our heart's flame, until you meld with us into God's mighty stream of Light, enabling you to then go forth into the world, where you'll shine as a beacon, and where all who encounter your radiance become magnetized from within to begin their transformation in consciousness and increased awareness of the multitudes of Beings who are here to help you and all life on Earth to evolve into higher and higher states of consciousness until all of Earth, together, explodes into her ascension of Light, and all are freed of Earth's density forever.

This is our role, this is our final goal to carry out on Earth, and then we will all, en masse, move up the spiral of evolution into the realm of Light and Love, and become who we truly are, living in a place of peace, beauty and prosperity, together as one cell in God's heart. So make this journey into Light with us, by opening your hearts to our existence and welcoming us into your life, so that we too, may guide you onto the steps of continual glory, where we step with you, side by side, on our path to God. So walk with us, hand in hand, and whenever you're weary, think of us holding you and supporting you as we all, as a planet, move closer and closer to our ascension. You are close, very close, and we are here to give you that extra push into the Light, where we all await your presence.

We bask in the Light of the Hollow Earth, where we have created a paradise within the womb of Mother Earth. And, we wish you, too, to experience this paradise along with us. We are now working closely with you, our brothers and sisters on the surface, and we cheer you on. I am Mikos, your friend from the past.

We Once Lived on Another Solar System

Greetings, my fellow travelers on Earth! Speaking to you today from inside the Hollow Earth, which is our home. We have been here for millions of years, slowly evolving ourselves into the God Beings that we are. Our evolution has made great strides due to the isolation of being wrapped up inside the womb of Mother Earth.

Ah, our lives have been spent in peace and bliss, due to our location. We exist here in peace and tranquility because of the proximity to the heartbeat of Mother Earth. The more deeply one goes into the Earth, the more deeply one feels the beat of the Earth. And the more one feels Her heartbeat, the more one resonates to her Goddess qualities. So this proximity has led Us, over the millennia, to our oneness with all life and to oujr joy of existence. All life knows this oneness, yet most of life has yet to feel it in their outer bodies.

As the heartbeat of Mother Earth reverberates through the Earth, it reaches the surface, where you can feel and experience it. However, in order to feel and resonate with this beat of life, you have to be in peace. Your outer bodies have to be in coordination and in synchronicity with each other, all vibrating at the same velocity and all feeling the grace of God and immersion in the oneness of Creation. When your bodies are at rest, at night, they resonate to the deep beat within them. You can only evolve when you are in a state of Peace. And this is why We, who are immersed in Earth's depths, have been able to evolve; because We have been in synchronicity with the beat of all life and with Our selves.

Once we were adrift in space, living on another solar system in the Milky Way Galaxy. At that time, there were what you today call "Star Wars". People were engaged in battles to control our section of the galaxy. These battles brought great destruction to planets and knocked solar systems off course. It was a dark time for our galaxy, and beings like ourselves yearned for peace to be restored so that we could continue our evolution. This is when we discovered the Earth.

We left our solar system and traveled here, which at the time was a planet little known outside its parameter. When We alighted on the surface, we were amazed and in awe of the beauty and tranquility of Earth. We explored the surface and found the open tunnels leading into the cavity inside. These were already existing tunnels from other civilizations, for the Earth is very old and her civilizations ancient.

All Planets Have Openings at Their North and South Poles We migrated through the poles and found our "nest" inside. The inside is so clean, so pure, and so peaceful, that from that time on we never left it.

Throughout the ages we have enlarged and expanded the tunnels leading to the Subterranean Cities and surface, as a means of travel for our inhabitants and yours. Although not too many surface travelers have used these tunnels, they exist for the future, when more of you and more of Us will intermingle and make the trip to visit each other. So the surface is dotted with tunnel entrances that you see on the map in this book, leading both to the Subterranean Cities and to Us. This is how it is on most planets in your galaxy, where geople travel freely to both the cradle and the rim, to exchange information and to learn on each other.

Your Earth has quite a history, going back into millennia of time. Unfortunately, its history isn't always peaceful, because once it was discovered, people fought great wars trying to control it and mine and remove its precious resources. So know that these times or raping the Earth are over with. These beings are no longer allowed entry to this sector of the Galaxy, which is steadily rising in Light, even as the waves lap the shores. The Light is flowing ceaselessly now, and bringing the tranquility and awareness that all surface dwellers yearn for.

We, here in the Hollow recesses of the Earth, have been calling for eons for more Light and for help from the Confederation of Planets to intercede to stop the influx of ravaging bands of ET's who have been scouring space to find planets that are rich in reserves like Earth. But today it is done. Know that the Confederation fully protects this sector, so that life can finally begin to evolve in peace.

Who Live in the Hollow Earth

We have easy access into the Inner Earth World through our tunnel system, which goes directly through the Earth's mantle and into the Inner Earth entryways, where we are greeted by our brothers and sisters upon our arrival. We are always going and coming, since we keep up a steady trade relation with them. We enjoy their beaches and oceans, and climb their mountains. It is a gloriously beautiful realm of Light and Purity, and truly invigorating to be there.

Know that the spiritual state of the Inner Earth Beings is very evolved compared to the surface dwellers. These Beings came from another solar system to populate the Inner Earth.

They never lived on the surface. Their home on this planet has always been in the inner recesses of Earth. They are, however, in contact with Beings on the surface, just as you are in contact with Adama in the mantle.

You, on the surface, are the direct descendants of roving bands of ET's, who created you to mine the Earth's resources. These Creator ET's don't reside on Earth at this time. However, you all have the same Spiritual potential as Inner Earth Beings. Your life on the surface in no way mirrors life in the Inner Earth. The only things on the surface that mirror life inwardly are the mountains and oceans and plains.

These Inner Earth Beings have your surface conditions fully monitored. They know all that transpires on Earth, just as we in the mantle know all through our computer network.

The great Inner Earth Beings know of your yearnings to live in the Inner Earth, where all is in a peaceful, harmonious state. They do consider surface folk their brothers and sisters who have not as yet evolved enough to reside with them in the "land of plenty". However, when you do reach a higher Spiritual state, then you, too, can live internally within Earth.

Space Portals and Travel

Our galaxy operates as one huge whole system, totally interconnected through an interstellar communication web. Through our portals located in the Library of Porthologos, we can contact anyone, or travel anywhere in our Universe and beyond.

Spaceports Inside the Earth

There are spaceports based inside Earth's interior, inside her mountains, beneath the oceans, inside the Hollow Earth cavity, that will take you on jaunts out to your solar system so you can witness first-hand the life on the planets around you. You will be in awe of Earth's majesty and in awe of God's creation - always humble and respectful as your experiences and beliefs drastically change into a knowingness that has up until now eluded you.

You are in for the thrill of your life. So just hold on as Earth goes through her changes, and know that you will be safe and cared for, no matter where your destination is. Every soul will be accounted for and every soul provided for in the great "play" called life on Earth. It is now the ending scene, and you are about to take your bows and leave the surface stage forever. You will reappear in another grand play, only this time you will play out your parts on a more conscious level, with more control of your lines and actions and in more control of your lives.

We in the Hollow Earth will be with you this time, helping and encouraging you to reach your fully conscious state, so that the whole planet can embark together on its next leg of the journey through life.

We Travel Freely Inside Our Globe

My dear friends of the Earth: I speak to you from the Great Cavern under your cities. This cavern spans the whole circumlerence of the center of the Earth. Our lives here are blessed with abundance in every way you can think of. Were you to let your imagination roam the Stars, all you can conceive of and more, we are blessed with. All we can imagine, we can manifest for ourselves. Such is the nature and natural law that exists everywhere you go in our Galaxy.

We are all Free Beings, free to travel and free to remain inside our cherished Earth. You may think our living space is cramped, but it is spacious, as our population is few compared to your billions. We travel freely inside our globe, needing no passports. Our means of travel is non-polluting, using only electromagnetic conveyances and crystal power. Your governments on the surface use these also, while keeping the secret well hidden from your populace. With all the rolling blackouts in California, soon your people will wake up to the unlimited supply of solar and wind and water/hydrogen power.

We are free to come and go as we please, and we often leave our homes for short trips to other star systems. We seldom visit your surface cities but prefer to view them on our computer screens. This is the safest and most comprehensive way to follow your activities worldwide.

We are always awake when you call to us, as we are attuned to your frequency and can instantly hear and feel your call. With over-brimming love in our hearts, we salute you for your dedication to our mission.

Through The Openings At The Poles

Our Spaceport is located inside the Hollow Earth, in direct alignment with the openings at the North and South Poles. We are not stuck on the Earth as you are but can leave whenever we desire. We are not limited in movement and can travel throughout the Universe at will. There are no physical constraints, for we apply the Universal Laws of Energy and use the already existing highways throughout the Universe. We can't get lost, for all is mapped out and all is in constant communication with all in existence. We just tap into this 'live' network that is always broadcasting and move through it effortlessly.

We are not isolated from the rest of life in our Universe - you are. We are not restricted in movement - you are.

As we are here in the Center of Earth's interior, you are here with us in consciousness. For consciousness is a 'place' - a place more solid than your physical places. So yes, you sit on the surface at your desk taking this dictation, but in consciousness, you are with us inside the Hollow Earth. You are literally in two places at once. Do you understand multidimensionalty now? Now that you are in both places simultaneously, we will show you around 'our place'. As you scan our landscape, you will 'see' the openings of the Holes at the Poles. These openings are wide enough for some Mother Ships to enter. You can 'see' the Spaceport, spread out for hundreds of miles in a circle interspersed with flowers, grasses, bushes, trees and waterfalls. It does not look like your barren, concrete airports, devoid of life; but rather like a garden with space shuttles and starships nestled peacefully inside our world.

We hardly know when they come and go, as they do not emit any harsh sounds, and we hardly detect any sound when they land or take off. They are in complete harmony with our love vibration and move in silence. We can visually see their movements as they gracefully fly in and out through the Poles. But this is the extent of it. There is no disturbance in sound or vibration, and there is no pollution and no destruction of our environment. This is quite a contrast from your surface airports, isn't it?

And, we never have "crashes," since every component of our craft is monitored by our aminoacid computers, and we detect and correct any problem immediately. Our technology is so far advanced from yours, for we've had the opportunity of peaceful living conditions to continuously develop it for millennia, without a break in our life spans. This is why your Immortality is so crucial. The longer you live in the same body, the more you can develop your talents and technologies, and the more you can create and refine things, rather than stopping and starting over again in each succeeding lifetime. All this stopping and starting over and over again gets you nowhere. You are continuously 'reinventing the wheel', and never moving beyond it. It is stagnation in evolution, getting you nowhere.

This is all ended now, as Mother/ Father God of this Universe has sent an edict that Earth has to move on, and can no longer hold the rest of the Galaxy back. All the other planets in your Solar System have already ascended, and it is only Earth that the whole Milky Way Galaxy has been waiting for. The laggards won't be able to hold Earth back any longer. From now on, all laggards will incarnate on an isolated planet where they won't be allowed to interfere with the evolution of a species, planet. Galaxy or Universe again. This is the edict that has been handed down from our Great Central Sun, Alpha and Omega.

Soon you will be feeling only bliss, as all negative forces and destructive entities will be leaving en masse through death, and exiting out of your Universe. The long suffering is over, and you will be free at last and will experience life as it was always meant to be experienced. You can feel this bliss now; feel the anticipation now, and bring it into your lives now - for it is already here, and will be getting stronger and stronger each day. Each day see your world through the eyes of Love and know in your heart that this is the future for Earth.

Our Portals Lead To All Star Systems

We are all gathered around me, as we step into our library and walk toward one of our many conference rooms, which are cozy and lined with the softest, supportive couches you've ever sat on. They are ergonomically structured to allow the life force to flow down our spines as we recline on them. The colors are brilliant in tone, and form a melody around our bodies.

There are many of us here in this room, as I dictate my message to you. They are holding the energy, so to speak, and flowing it toward you as you sit at your computer.

Yes, our Library is a multi-dimensional portal and way-station for travelers around the galaxy. Beings come here from all dimensions and universes to witness the wonders of creation, that unfold when they step into the vast portals that transport them into realms beyond their imagination. It is such a wondrous place to be, and the wonders are limitless. It takes infinity to experience them all, as life and learning go on indefinitely and forever. There is always more to learn and more places to go. This is what awaits you all when you visit us in the Hollow Earth and are invited to enter the Library of Porthologos. It is written on your cosmic passport, that once you are here in our realm, your entry to the portals is assured. It is the opening to all of creation, and it is located right here in the center of your Earth. What a wondrous journey awaits you. We keep our doors open to all who come, and once you are here, you come with a divine ticket to enter. Your ticket of admittance is encoded in your DNA. You can also come at night, in your sleep state, for a preview of what lies ahead of you when you do enter in your physical body. This will help you acclimate to the real 'show' so that when you finally do enter our realm it will seem so familiar to you, and you'll feel that you've been here before.

There are portals leading to all Star Systems in our, just waiting for you to explore. You will become a Star Traveler, learning from each Star System as you make your way around the galaxy. This is a never-ending journey of course, because life goes on forever, and exploration goes on forever as our universes keep expanding exponentially into infinity.

This gives us something to do. For life is about 'doing'. We need something to do in life in order to bring us the experiences for our soul growth. And the Creator supplies more universes than we could ever possibly explore in all of infinity, which just keeps unfolding and unfolding as our experiences increase. Can you imagine this? Your stepping down into our realm is the first step of your exploration out of limitation and density and into the unlimited vastness of experience and space. Our portals offer you all this and more, along with the comforts of home as you travel back and forth.

We have been here for eons, and yet have explored only a fraction of our galaxy. . .and there are billions of galaxies in billions of universes just waiting for us all to visit. Your life will forevermore be filled with excitement, and you'll never again find yourself saying: "What shall we do today?"

Portal to the Sun

We are attired in our finest clothing to meet with you this morning. The stin is shining overhead, and we are standing on the steps of the Library of Porthologos about to enter this vast portal, and take you inside with us. Walk with us now, as we surround your etheric body with our light and love. We usher you into our great entrance hall, that is lined in beauty and light and that sings to our souls. We will walk but a few steps to one of the moving staircases that will take us to a portal where we can witness the vastness of our galaxy. It is the galactic portal to this galaxy, and from there we can choose the destination where we desire to go. It is the fastest means of travel. No ticket or luggage is required, just our hearts intention. So here we go. We stand beside the entrance to this portal, where we form our destination desire, before entering. Are you ready? Let's go to the center of our Sun, where you have many friends and lineage waiting for you. Ok? Let's step in now, focus on the Sun, and we are there. It is that quick. See around you the brilliant light and feel the love that permeates your body and soul, and hear the choruses of angelic music. Sananda is here, and he greets you in his loving embrace and covers you with his light. We start walking now toward the community above the horizon, just a few steps away. It is nestled in hues of color and warmth and the houses are all different shades of vibrant colors. People are all outdoors, tending their fields and visiting and just lounging around. All are receptive and joyous to greet us, and knew of our intention of coming.

These beings have all made their passage from Earth and given the opportunity to live here on the Sun for as long as they like. They passed their Earthly tests with flying colors, and earned this opportunity to reside here in the great love and light of our Sun, which is a planet also, but a planet of such great light that it lights your whole solar system. This is what the Earth is turning into. It is turning into a great sun star that in turn will give life and light and warmth to other planets in its solar system. And it, too, has earned this. As the Earth moves up in consciousness, she will ignite into a blazing sun star, and take all those souls who are attuned to her, with her. The other souls will be taken to another planet to continue along in their evolution, until they too, reach such states of light, that they, too, will have this opportunity to relocate into a higher frequency realm.

We now walk back to the portal and focus on returning to the Library of Porthologos, where we now again are standing on the steps. We all hug you goodbye, and thank you with the fullness of our hearts for making this journey with us today. It is indeed a grand celebration when we meet with you for these sessions. We bid you adieu.

Free Energy and Abundance

The Earth provides FREE Sources of ENERGY

We speak to you today on behalf of our Beloved Mother Earth, in whose womb we dwell. All our lives we have lived in peace and abundance, always knowing that all we could ever need would be provided for us. This is the responsibility of a mother. This is the purpose of our Earth - to provide abundance to all life living upon her. We have accepted all that the Earth has given to us, in gratefulness, without ever taking more than we need. All of us understand the great Universal Laws of Life, and all of us live by them. These laws are simple and logical, and state that, whatever you sow, you reap. We live our lives in harmony with our Earth Mother, and in return she supplies us with all we need. It is a quite simple law to follow, and reaps great riches.

The Earth is a self-sufficient planet, supplying all that life needs from within her own body. She is ever replenishing herself, and ever replenishing her harvests.

You are taking more from the Earth than you need, since energy is free, but you insist on using fossil fuels instead of cultivating the free sources of energy that are plentiful to everyone on the planet. This is depleting the Earth of her natural resources, which in reality function as parts of her body. When these parts are continually mined and depleted, the Earth will not be able to function. Just as if someone mined your heart center, you would not be able to survive.

Every part of Earth serves a function, and must function in order for her to survive. There's a world of free energy out there, just waiting for you to harness. There's electromagnetic energy, wind, solar, tidal and others that you haven't even discovered yet. This cold winter is giving you a great opportunity to develop other forms of fuel to heat your homes and run your industries. How fortunate prices for gas are soaring, for its purpose is to bring to your attention the availability of other energy sources that are FREE. Why pay a utility company for what the Earth provides for free?

The Earth has always given you more than you need, but in your greed you have stripped her of her resources of gold and uranium and other metals, which are her life force. Soon your people will wake up to the unlimited supply of solar and water/ hydrogen power.

We in the Hollow Earth never pay for anything; for all the Earth gives us is free and this freedom allows us to cultivate our creativity and spirituality and relationships which results in 'Heaven on Earth' for us.

Harmony Restores the Flow of Abundance

We've been waiting patiently for you on the steps of the Library of Porthologos, in the stillness of the Hollow Earth, where all is serene. Today we greet you in the Light of the One Creator, the Creator of all, no matter where you live on this Earth. We were all designed by the Great Designer and here to fulfill the divine plan for Earth.

Today we will talk about life inside the globe, and how it glorifies our existence in physical form. Everything here is in a heightened state of evolution, and everything here responds immediately to our thoughts. We command the elements, and the elements work with us, not against us, to bring us our perfect climate and perfect environment. Everything responds to everything, and together creates a synergy of resonating melodies that uplift and nourish our souls. We are constantly being fed by the vibrations of all life around us, restoring ourselves continuously and fully with the great life force necessary for our existence in immortality.

You on the surface are diametrically opposed to everything and everyone, sheltered in your own realities of separateness, and not heeding the forces of nature who are there to work with you, but whom you deem necessary to destroy and plunder. This is a great travesty of life, and as a result your environment is crashing at a rapid pace. The most important lesson to learn in this lifetime, is to live in harmony with all life, all people, all of nature. Once humanity learns this, then the great forces of abundance will flow to everyone, and suddenly everyone will have everything they could ever need. It is all available to you right now, once harmony is restored on the surface.

But you who read these messages know this, and are carrying vast amounts of Light. And it is your Light that is touching the garments of all you come in contact with and raising the vibration of the planet. It is your Light that is blazing through the density, clearing the haze of distortion so that humanity can, once again, see clearly.

Technology

Greetings from the Hollow Earth. I am Mikos, your friend from inside the Earth. Thank you for opening your computer to talk to us. We are all gathered around me, as I dictate this message to you from underground. We are also gathered around you, in your office, as you type this dictation. We are holding the energy, and the Light of protection around you, as you sit at your computer.

Today we will talk about the technology inside the Earth. We are all technologically advanced inside the Earth, and all of our technology is used for construction, not destruction, of our civilizations. We use all our technology for only the highest purposes to advance our civilizations and improve our living conditions. We already live very well, and we are always refining our living mode, as each step upwards is another step to God. We are always advancing in everything we do, whether it is for ourselves or for others.

On the surface, your technology is used to make and amass weapons of destruction, to be used on the human race. But remember, when you use weapons of destruction on the human race, you are also eradicating the other species that share this planet with you, and you are also upsetting their habitants, leaving them homeless too. Have you ever thought about this?

Your karma for destruction is great, because it is not only for humans, but the elemental kingdom and animal kingdom and the trees that you maim and obliterate when you use your weapons of mass destruction.

You have reversed the purpose for developing technology in the first place. Its purpose is to advance living conditions and create ease and plenty for everyone, not to harm and destroy each other and the land. This is a gross misuse of God's technology that was given to you to improve your lives and experiment with different ways of living, not to destroy the very lives that you were meant to improve. There is a great misunderstanding here, that we wish to clarify for you. Although most of the Earth's population is loving and yearns only for peace, there are still thousands who wish to control the population of Earth, including all her resources. They do this through war and threats.

The only way to advance is through the heart center, where love from God flows to each and every one of us. Here, in the Hollow Earth, our hearts are always open, and always receiving the love that is pouring in from God. Love is all we feel. It is this same love that is also pouring into your hearts on the surface. All you have to do is open to receive it, and you will feel its wonders in every thought you think and every emotion you feel. You will be tuned into God, even though your feet still touch the Earth.

Electrons Remain Intact In Our Water

We don't use the same technology to bring our water to us as you on the surface do. Our 'pipes' operate differently so that when our water flows through them, the electrons remain intact. When water flows through the pipes on the surface, the electrons spin off, resulting in the loss of life force. So you drink 'dead' water, due to the way water spirals through your pipes. This does not occur in the Hollow Earth or Subterranean Cities, because we know how to flow water to keep its electrons intact and protect its life force. So the water we drink is alive. It is living consciousness.

When we emerge and come to the surface, we will bring our equipment with us, connected to the Hollow Earth oceans, and deliver water to you that you've never tasted before; water that invigorates your spirit, renews your cells and rebuilds your body. We will clean all your oceans and streams, and show you how to harness the life force and bring it right into your homes.

We Store Our Records On Telonium Plates

I am talking to you from my office in the Library of Porthologos, where I transcribe and prepare all ancient, current and future records for our Telonium plates. Telonium is an ancient and eternal kind of metal that lasts forever and never shown any signs of decay. It is the perfect material to store our records on. This process of storage is quite a creative one, and it's a joy to indulge ourselves in the creation process of preserving all of Earth's records, along with all the records in our Universe. It is a process of extreme creativity, not like working in a surface copy shop or the mundane repetition of factory work.

Uncovering Our Existence

We Are the Diamonds and You Are the Miners.

We are here, embedded in the Earth's core, like sparkling diamonds buried in a mine. You can only reach us by uncovering the stratums of Earth that cover up our Light. You do this by leering yourself of all impurities and emotional blocks, so that your vision is clear and focused. Once your sight is attuned to our frequency, you will see us clearly, sparkling under the Inner Central Sun of the inner sphere of Earth. For though you do not as yet 'see' us, you can feel our existence under you by connecting with us in consciousness. You will physically feel your vibratory rate increase, and your crown chakra will bubble and pulse. This is a physical manifestation of your connection to us.

Yes, we are the diamonds buried inside the Earth, and you are the miners about to reach down and uncover our existence below you. Soon, we will receive the directive from the Confederation of Planets, to swing open the Tunnel Entrances for you to physically enter our realm and explore the inside cavity of Earth.

Be assured that we will have guides leading you through the tunnels, seating you on our electromagnetic vehicles and escorting you to our cities where you will be cheered and congratulated for reaching the frequency where you can visit us at last. When this occurs, it will be the sign that the Earth's ascension is imminent. What a glorious day this will be. For not only we and you will celebrate, but the Whole Universe will be applauding your emergence out of density; signaling to all that our Whole Galaxy is now prepared to move, as a whole, to a higher octave of existence.

For remember, that with unity consciousness, we all accelerate as one - one universe accelerating on her course through eternity, through the ever-expanding light of god, of all that is.

The Earth herself is a diamond, a multifaceted gem radiating the brilliance of God's Eternal Light. It is only surface folk, separated by the veils of density, who are blinded to the brilliance surrounding titiem. The brilliance is within your souls, within the Earth, and within all life everywhere. Just turn your eyesight inwardly, feel your connection to All That Is, and your Inner World will light up and resonate to the diamond you are. Through this resonance, all of Earth will open up to you in all its glory and splendor, and you will see all and know all. The world of Light is within your soul. It is self-lit by the Source of All and sustained eternally.

The merging of our two civilizations will signal the accomplishment of the Divine Plan on Earth, and you will be free to evolve up the Spiral of Evolution at long last, without the impediments and blockages and obstacles and density of the last 12 million years. So rise with us in consciousness, as we merge into One Diamond of Sparkling Light wrapped around and through our entire planet. I am Mikos of the Diamond Light.

Huge, Carved-Out Cavity

The Library of Porthologos is vast and round, situated within the inside of the Hollow Earth cavity. We are in a huge, carved-out cavity. We are not out in the open as you might imagine. Mother Earth keeps her inner grounds pristine by providing living space within her interior body and not out in the open spaces.

Our inner caverns are perfectly suited to our living style and when we want to swim in the oceans or climb the mountains, it is but a short trip to the center of the Hollow Earth cavity in our electromagnetic vehicles that levitate through the vast tunnel system in just minutes of your time. You will all experience this soon, as the time of our emergence will bring us to you and we will escort you to our homes within the Earth. All is lit up in the softest and clearest of light, and the temperatures are perfectly suited to our health and strength.

All our lives we've waited for this moment to connect with you on the surface, and now it is here. Our hearts are brimming over with love for all our lost brothers and sisters, and we yearn to connect to each and every one of you again. Our hearts are one.

Our Haven Underground

There are so many Catharians gathered around me, Mikos, as I dictate this message to you. We are out on the grounds that surround the great Library of Porthologos. We are sitting on grass that is as soft as a cushion, breathing in the fragrant, oxygen-filled air that keeps us eternally young and vibrant. This pure air is "nectar" to our lungs, and keeps our bodies free from disease.

The oxygen on the surface has reached such low levels that you are being oxygen starved, which opens the way for pathogens to invade your body. We, here in the Hollow Earth, breathe clean, pure air, and drink the purest of water, which is still as pure as the day Earth was created. We are so fortunate to be living in this haven under the ground. We sit here, propped up comfortably on our pillows and stools, just breathing in the air and smelling the scents of the enormous flowers blooming all around us. This is a wonderland of beauty, and this beauty is reflected in our souls.

Our bodies respond to our environment, and out-picture what surrounds us. And what surrounds us is magnificent to behold. We are surrounded by trees and flowers that emanate strength and health, and we in turn feel this strength and health, and our bodies conform to this picture. So our bodies mirror our surroundings. They mirror the perfection of our environment. We, in turn, mirror perfection back thus completing the cycle of perfection that is never ending. Because of this perfect cycle, our bodies can remain in a perpetual state of perfection, never sickening, nor aging, nor dying. It is a closed cycle of perfection.

It is noon here now, and we bask in the full spectrum light of our Inner Central Sun, as it hangs in our "sky." Our sky is the very center of the Hollow Globe, and our sun doesn't move, as your sun appears to. Ours just hangs there, "dead center", held by the forces of gravity pulling around its circumference so that it is perfectly balanced and remains in place.

The inside of the Earth is concave, and spirals up and across and around us. So our picture of "heaven" is from a different perspective or angle than yours. You look straight "up", and we look "around" us. So today, as always, the sun is shining down upon our gathering here on the Library Grounds. Our work here in the Library is not work as you term it, but joy to our hearts.

We do what we love, and we do it in leisure. We have no time clocks to punch, and no time clocks to tell us when to stop. We each know what we want to accomplish each day, and we stay as long as we want or until we complete our work. However, we don't set long hours the way you do on the surface. Our workday is short compared to yours. In terms of hours, our workday is less than half the hours of your work day. So should we want to work "overtime", we have the flexibility of doing so without it infringing on the other areas of our lives. And our lives remain always balanced, because our schedules allow us the time to do so many other things each and every day, above and beyond the hours we spend on our "jobs".

We live perfectly balanced lives of ease and comfort, and have created everything we need to develop our talents, expand our minds, and strengthen our bodies. We have music and dance conservatories and theatres everywhere. We are always dancing and singing together, fine tuning our talents and evolving them to do more and more creative things.

Our lives are filled with creativity, and we delight in what we create. For what we create is shared with all, so that we all benefit from each other's talents and abilities. We all teach each other and we all learn from each other. We thrive on cooperation, we thrive on sharing, and we thrive on giving as much as we can to each other, which means that we end up having all that we've all created. So our gifts are multiplied — our blessings are multiplied — and we reap the abundance of our civilization underground. Nothing is hoarded or "owned", as you do on the surface, for it's not necessary, nor even logical, when you understand that we are all a part of the Earth, and therefore everything belongs to everyone, and yet nothing is owned by anyone, because everything is free for everyone to use.

Sharing is the key not owning. Just change your words and you will change your ways. And changing the way you do things will change your lives — and will bring them back into balance, so that you, too, will have the leisure to develop your creativity and talents and explore the Earth, rather than devour her. For once you explore the intricacies and beauty and magic of Nature, you cannot abhor and destroy her, you can only emulate and love her, and know beyond a doubt that she is you, and you are her. For whatever you destroy outside yourself, you destroy within yourself, for Nature out-pictures you, as much as you out-picture Nature.

Just look around you at the devastation of Earth's forests and oceans, and it will show you the parts of yourself that you are destroying inside your very own bodies. The Earthquakes that are becoming so prevalent on the surface are now surfacing within your very own emotional and physical bodies.

Everything you do to the Earth, you do to yourself. Remember, there is only one consciousness. You and We are part of the one consciousness. As you destroy a part of the one, the other parts are affected.

You are not separate from the Earth. You are the Earth; you just don't know it yet. But as you wake up from your deep slumber of millions of Earth years, you will remember the connectiveness of all life, and how the health of one is connected to the health of all. Surface humans cannot survive if they destroy their surroundings and wage wars on their own species, just because they live on different parts of the planet.

We, here in Porthologos, are so grateful to each blade of grass, to each petal on a flower, to each leaf on a tree. For the harmony we feel is the same harmony that the flowers and trees feel, and which enables us to grow in stature and accounts for the enormity in size of our trees, which tower above the ground like your skyscrapers, because nothing is holding them back.

They and we are free to grow in size, free to expand ourselves, because everything is in a state of expansion, not contraction as you witness and experience on the surface.

When you are "open" to life, you can only expand. When you are in struggle and lack and fear, you can only close down and diminish your stature, for fear of being seen or fear of standing out among others. You squelch your power, squelch your intuition, squelch your feelings, trying to fit into the mold of the lowest common denominator of the people around you. This stunts not only your physical growth but your soul growth as well. When you open to the fact that you and the Universe are one, you will awaken to all that you are and begin to expand your horizons and literally grow in size — height and width.

Your mind and body are connected. If you think small, you grow small. If you think life only exists on Earth's surface and nowhere else, then you've shortened yourself, which shortens your physical height, just as your thoughts have shortened your vision. Expand your thoughts, and you expand your world; expand your world, and your body responds in spurts of growth and renewal.

If you only knew all that you are, you would be living like Kings and Queens, in palaces of gold, not on dirty, littered city streets. You've dethroned yourself, and you don't even know it.

Wake Up, Surface Dwellers! For if you don't, the earthquakes within your souls will blast you back into consciousness of who you are — and that might mean the devastation of your current living conditions being turned to rubble.

Although it's hard work to dig yourself out of an earthquake, once you're free of its rubble and you see that everything you "owned" is gone, you will awaken with the shock and realize that all you have is yourself. Suddenly, from within the depths of your Being, you find the strength and wisdom that was buried inside you. earthquakes clear density, so sight is restored and vision returned, enabling you to see and be all that you truly are.

Our vision has always been clear, since density does not cloud our vision underground. We see clear and far, because nothing obstructs our vision. We can see out among the Stars, even though we're under the ground, because nothing impedes our sight.

When you clear yourselves of all belief systems and negative thoughts and negative feelings, you too will feel the clarity and harmony within yourselves, and will be able to see all that has been kept from you by your governments. You will be able to "see through" all their deceit. And the truth about life on other planets and life within the Earth will shine through your eyes and be fully exposed to all.

We are still sitting here beneath our sun as I bring this dictation to its end. We thank you for taking our message.

Time, Telepathy, and Consciousness

The Amount of Time You Have in Each Day Is Determined by Your Level of Consciousness.

Earth is out of time with the rest of the Universe, in order for her evolutions to learn the lessons of their souls. Time operates differently here on Earth's surface, for its peoples need to repeat life's lessons over and over again until they are learned and mastered. That is why you have the concept of past, present and future - to give your evolving human species the time they need to learn their lessons and pass the tests necessary for mastery. So Earth time plays an important factor in evolution.

When a planet evolves and is in the Ascended State, there is no more time, for from this higher perspective of consciousness you can see into Eternity - and can feel the oneness of all time simultaneously. You indeed experience your multidimensionality, which is experiencing all states of consciousness and all time and places at once. There are no longer any demarcations or divisions or separateness. All is ONE, and all is simultaneous.

As Earth and all life on her surface evolve in consciousness, time compresses. It becomes less and less, which is a sign that humans are evolving in consciousness. This results in less and less time, until you reach the point in your consciousness when you're no longer "in" time - you've moved out of it into the Ascended State.

As you move higher and higher in your awareness of yourself and all of Earth, you will find that the days speed by, even the minutes and hours fly by, and before you know it, morning turns into night before you've accomplished even half of what you used to be able to accomplish.

Time is actually becoming elusive. You can't hold onto it any longer. The denser an evolution is, the more time there is, and the days appear longer. The higher the vibration of a species, the shorter the day appears, as they are actually connecting with "Cosmic Consciousness", which is a state of multidimensionality where "no time" exists. Everything just "is".

As time further collapses, you will move into the multidimensionality that you are, and experience "All That Is" profoundly. You will see and feel the Oneness of all Creation, and how all life is intertwined and interconnected. This is what humanity is here to learn. But up until now Earth's density has been so thick that each person has felt separated and alone, and cut off from others. Each person has felt separated by time and space - which in actuality does not exist. It only exists on "evolving" planets so that its species does not get sidetracked and can focus in on what it came here to do.

Time flow has nothing to do with age. It does not speed up when you are older. It only speeds up when you are wiser and have "grown" in consciousness and wisdom. Therefore, if you equate age with wisdom and illumination, then indeed you could say that as you age, time speeds up. But for those who don't evolve in consciousness during their life spans, then time seems interminably long and drawn out for them. They could say that "time gets slower" as they get older. So you see, it's your own perspective, your own rate of evolution that determines times length - and determines the length of each of your own days. You all have different day lengths and different amounts of time, determined by your state of consciousness. So as your consciousness expands, your minutes and hours decrease in reverse ratio; until you're no longer in a time zone, but in an Ascended State of Enlightenment, where there's no time, no space - only the Oneness of all Creation.

This is what we experience in the Hollow Earth. We feel the ONENESS and ETERNITY of existence. And this Oneness and Eternity is what you are beginning to experience on the surface, in small increments, as the Light of the Creator is pouring onto Earth and causing your consciousness to expand with the illumination of God's Light.

We don't feel the "crunch" of time, as you would say. We feel only the Eternal flow of life ebbing through us, which brings us peace and contentment in every "moment" of our day. We don't even have clocks (as you do and rely upon). We count time in a much different, cosmic way, that's in synchronicity with the whole cosmos. Because we are part of the cosmos, and function as part of the cosmos, we are on "cosmic time" - which is much different from surface time.

As the Light is rapidly illuminating the Earth, soon your consciousness will reach into cosmic time, and you will find us waiting for you there, which is right here - in the NOW. We wish you a speedy journey in consciousness.

You Have More Than Five Senses

We come here to meet with you to give you messages to take to your people who are above ground. It is so very important that the people here on Earth know who we are and that we are here. Our existence is crucial to your existence. You are much wiser now as a species and will more easily accept us when we physically contact you now.

This Hollow Globe you live above was meant for all to partake in, was meant for all to explore, was meant for all to realize how magnificent the God within is. For it is the God within your being who has created all of this, and it is the God within your being who wants to experience all of this. But first you have to recognize its existence and recognize that things do exist beyond your five senses, beyond that which you call sight and sound and location, for you don't need to be able to see something in order for it to exist. Its existence is independent of your actual physical sight.

In actuality, you will have many more than the five senses. In actuality, you are all multidimensional beings, who are here to discover the other senses within your multidimensionality. And when you discover your extra senses, you will discover the Universe. You won't need books to learn from anymore, for all of the learning will take place within you. You'll be able to travel any place you desire and learn from the actual experience of going there.

Books will become obsolete, for the real place of knowledge is within. As Jesus said, know yourself, and you will know everything. For you are the source of everything, you are where everything is stored; you only need to learn how to access the Living Library within your very being, within your very body, within your Temple.

Marvelous things await you as you raise yourself in consciousness and raise yourselves to higher frequencies of Light Vibrations. The higher you vibrate, the more you can access, and the more you can access, the more of yourself you will know. All knowledge is within you, and you are within all, and it is quite simple to access it once you've moved up your vibration to the necessary frequency where suddenly all becomes available to you and all becomes a gift from the Grand Creator of All That Is.

So the purpose of life is to move up in vibration until you are where we are, until all you can see is pure essence of life, the pure essence of all that is, and this pure essence is the Nirvana that you all have been looking for. The pure essence of God, which dwells in each of us, is the essence that creates the Worlds Within the Worlds.

You are now reaching the point in your evolution where it will be very easy for you to access all that is, to access the greatness of your body cells, and once again unite with us in consciousness. And once this uniting takes place, you will greatly benefit from all that we have learned over these eons of time. For we have been able to put our consciousness to work, so to speak, to create a Nirvana inside the Globe of Mother Earth.

Mother Earth knows of the existence of all of her children; she knows where each of us is, how each of us is, and where we're all going on our path to destiny. As you raise yourself in consciousness, you will also be able to check in with Mother Earth and she will tell you how you're doing as your consciousness registers within her, as the Light of your being is known by her, as all that you do and all that you say is heard by her. So you are, indeed, fully equipped to begin your journey into the bright light of a new Earth, into the bright light of the new world, where we all excitedly await your return.

There Is No Delay in Telepathic Transmissions

All are standing around me as I relay this dictated message to you that you are receiving hundreds of miles above us.

There is no delay in telepathic transmissions. You hear what I say instantaneously, at the exact moment that I say it. It is quite a miraculous way to communicate, and also quite a natural way, as you will soon all realize as you raise yourself in harmony with us; for it is in this harmonious mode that telepathic communication can take place. For it is the harmony of our beings that meld and merge into one another so that we can talk to each other whenever we so desire.

Open yourselves up to the existence of other life existing beside you on your home planet and you will be able to explore all the wonders that truly do exist inside this globe you call Earth. She is a wonder in herself, our Earth, and the more you come to know her, the more you come to know yourself and the more you come to know all life. For the existence of all life can be accessed by you as you move yourself up into higher frequencies of consciousness. We can see and hear all of you who live above us, as you are all very closely monitored by us. We know of all that takes place on the surface through our vision and through our computer system, where all on Earth is monitored closely and where our emissaries come in and out of our habitat, bringing us news and also relaying information to surface dwellers.

Our emissaries are in contact with many surface dwellers who work with us in the dissemination of information regarding the conditions on the surface. We do have quite a system going that will greatly surprise you. Until that time approaches when you will be able to visit, I will be speaking directly to you, exchanging information with you from the Hollow Earth that you can access within your very own beings.

So do connect with us in consciousness, as we are all here and all very eager to return your reply. We will speak to all who consciously connect with us in sincerity of heart, for it is our greatest wish to connect with you and help you through these times where you will soon be aware of all life on Earth and where we all will recognize all of us as ONE.

Telepathy

You have been gifted beyond measure with talents and intelligence that are now surfacing. Many of you are regaining your gifts that were hidden from your sight. One of these is telepathy.

You are all telepathic, and you can all converse with Us. You are just now beginning to realize how gifted humans really are. So gifted, that in fact you could actually do everything that we do, because we were once you.

We once went through all that you are now experiencing. But with our entry into the cavity of Earth, we were destined to evolve, just as you are destined to evolve as the Earth's frequency speeds up. Your innate gifts will shine through and you will rejoice at your capabilities. Once you reach a certain frequency, your consciousness will burst through the density and you will see all and know all, and we will be here with you at last, enfolding you in our love.

You Are the Knower of All.

You are the ONE component necessary for ALL to exist.

Your existence is the primary factor for the existence of the Universe.

Without you, each and every one of you there could be no life.

You are all an integral part in the design and not one of you is superfluous.

Know how important you are.

Know how necessary you each are.

For without each one of you, there is nothing.

Your existence makes up the substance of ALL THAT IS.

You are each the necessary ingredient.

That makes the Universe work with precision.

Cures for Pollution and Diseases

We have the answers to all your pollution problems that your greedy politicians and secret governments have created. And once we have surfaced, we will put our technologies into operation to solve all your pollution problems and all your health problems. Once your pollution is cleared up, your diseases will vanish. For your diseases are only caused by you polluting your air, water and foods. It's so simple, if you would but grasp the truth of it.

Here in the Hollow Earth, we never pollute anything, as this word does not even exist for us.

We live in complete harmony with our surroundings and our people know that we are all a part of each other. We would never do anything to harm one another, nor would the thought ever cross our minds. We feel only love for each other, and love for our surroundings and love for our Mother Earth. It is this love component that you are missing on the surface. You've put everything before love, and lost your sight and lost your way. It is now time to return love back into your lives, and it will solve all your surface problems in the quick of a winlc.

We follow your thoughts from below, and send our love to intercept your thoughts from above, hoping to gently guide you into a state of pure love in your thinking process. For when your thoughts become the beacons of pure love radiating out from you, you will bring the peace and harmony to your surface civilizations that you all desire so much.

The Cure For All Diseases Already Exists

Today is a celebration for Us in the Hollow Earth. We are celebrating our climb into Light, for we've reached a demarcation, a certain level of growth that we have been working toward for some time now. It's a whole new way of looking at life; it's reaching another step on the ladder of evolution and it's an exciting time for us as we embark on experiencing this whole new perspective to life. Each level we reach is an eye-opener, and we wonder how we couldn't have seen this before. This is similar to your eye openers on the surface, as it is the way all life evolves. More and more of the 'unseen' becomes the 'seen'.

This is now happening to you also on the surface. More and more is being revealed to you on your newscasts and newspaper. This is an exciting time for you too, for that which is being revealed has already been known for decades, but kept hidden from the public. With all the light reaching the Earth, the secrets are being exposed because Light exposes everything. It is only darkness that "covers up." You are in for the 'ride of your life', as everything that has been kept from you will suddenly come out in the media. What a 'shake up' will soon occur.

The medical groups, corporations and governments that have been covering up the cures to diseases and then spending billions of your tax dollars to 'find' cures, will be exposed. These groups caused the diseases in the first place, and could have easily stopped them years ago.

Instead, they've used disease as a profit generator - a way to make billions of dollars at the expense of a suffering humanity. All the diseases have been caused by corporations and governments polluting your air, water and food with chemicals, herbicides, pesticides, fertilizers, biological germs, and you name it; along with destroying the rainforests and cetaceans. All they have to do is stop this pollution to rid the Earth of its effects. But it's their greed, at the expense of humanity and Earth that has prevailed. For they will all be exposed for exactly who they are: profiteers in the worse sense, whose goal has been to rape and destroy a planet and its people.

We have no diseases in the Hollow Earth because we grow everything organically, and know and revere the connection between our Earth and our lives. We know we are part of the Earth and whatever we do to her we do to ourselves. As more and more of humanity reconnect themselves to Nature, they will understand how to eliminate all diseases and destruction on Earth.

This is what Light does. It opens your eyes and reconnects you to the Source of all Creation, so you can again live your lives in peace and plenty and perfect health.

So join us in consciousness, as we gently lead you to Nirvana, where you will dwell with us at last.

Protect your Newborn from Inoculations

There's a whole new Earth being birthed, and all souls are now being born with telepathy and clairvoyance and great wisdom. This is why your government has its inoculation system in place in your hospitals. These inoculations jam the high frequencies of the newborn and prevent their accessing the divine gifts that they are innately endowed with. This is the purpose of these 'mandatory' inoculations - they are to keep the Light of your newborn off the planet.

So remember dear ones, not to give into the fear of your hospitals or your media, and stand in your own Light of Wisdom, of knowing that nothing can harm your newborn, as they are divinely endowed and protected from the illnesses of this planet. They come fully equipped to withstand all adverse conditions and nothing administered to them by your hospitals or doctors can protect them - it will only deflect their health from them. So protect your newborns by knowing that they are already protected from within their own DNA, and no outside antidote or inoculation can benefit them in any way.

They, too, are the Angels incarnating on Earth and being born to you at this time to bring more and more Light to Earth. As Earth's frequency of Light increases, we cheer from below, knowing that our emergence is indeed imminent. We leave now in the Light and Love of our Creator.

A Great Dispensation Has Just Been Granted

Greetings from the Library of Porthologos inside the Earth's interior. We come today to talk about the Angels on Earth and their work with humanity. These are great Beings of Light from many Star Systems that are visiting your Earth, and staying to help bring in the great waves of Light that are descending onto your planet. These Beings are most known to you as Angels - God's helpers in the evolution of mankind. These Beings sweep your planet with their light and wisdom, encapsulate the dark spots until the darkness fades back into Light again. The Angels are the bringers of all that is good, and they are here. And you, our dear Light workers, are these Angels. You are these great Beings who have come from afar, to help Earth and humanity, and now it is your turn to be helped. A great dispensation has just been granted to all the Light workers on Earth, allowing the Host of Heaven to intervene to completely and totally heal your physical bodies, so that you can withstand the coming climatic and Earth changes looming on the horizon of your planet. You have all called for help, you are always calling for the healing of your bodies, and now this help has been granted.

In a magnificent turn of events, this dispensation was unanimously approved by the whole company of heaven, and Mother/ Father God of this Universe, in gratefulness for the dedication and sacrifice of all the Light workers on Earth - and it is time. Time to heal all aspects of yourself and time to manifest your physical strength, health, mental acuity and emotional balance. This is the gift of Heaven to its 'Ground Crew". As the days and weeks go on, you will find yourself getting stronger and stronger, and all the old pains falling by the wayside. You will see and feel events clearer and clearer and come more into focus with the unseen world around you. This is truly an unprecedented gift, and it is yours.

Now, dear Light workers, live each day fully, in the presence of the 'now', and know that tomorrow is in God's hands, and have nothing to fear, for the Divine Plan is already accomplished and this is just the last 'play-off of the game. All is being readied for the great 'liftoff into higher realms of light that are waiting your entry. You have much to look forward to as you leave your old world behind and enter the new. So gird yourself with the steel of your determination and know that all that is of the Light has a glorious future and it is just a breath away - just waiting for the next deep in-breath from God.

Here in the Library of Porthologos, we have always maintained our health, strength and youthfulness inside the protective cover of the Earth's mantle. You, too, will soon be able to accomplish the same physical feats and will have the same endurance as we. For we don't get tired or sick or angry or worried, and neither, now, shall you. For these qualities are not of life - they are of illusion and mis-creation and darkness - and are not part of a life supporting system. Your current system does not support life; hence you have sickness, fear and death. It has been decreed that these systems can no longer exist, and will be confined and quarantined like a sick patient, in a separate room. Only this time, all the sick patients will be in a ward by themselves, so they don't infect the others. No one again will nave to suffer from their control and destructive contamination.

Evolution is the Solution

Now we will talk about the World Trade Center and the atrocities. As you can see, 911 is the emergency number for help. On this date was a call for help from the people of the world against all terrorists. This emergency call was a shout to heaven, and all in our galaxy and beyond heard your cries for help. It was a grand unification of souls, unified in your distress and pain, and calling to God for help and for freedom from tyranny.

Your people are united on the soul level, each one wanting peace to be able to live out your life in freedom. There was a great divine response to the tragedy. This was not a setback for the Light, but instead, a grand opening for us to become part of your conscious life and to intervene even more in the affairs of Earth to bring the peace you all strive for.

Out of every tragedy comes a grand awakening, and millions more have awakened to the Light as a result of this. The dark forces are actually working for us when they scheme to perpetrate such heinous acts of violence. It wakes people from their comfort zones of slumber and they start calling on God at last and reconnect their phone line to the Divine Creator of ALL.

So look at this as another step that humanity has taken towards the Light that reaches you all from heaven. For once humanity connects again to the Light, it will flow forth to the Earth like a waterfall rushes to the ground, bathing all and soaking you through to your core with Light. It is an immersion into Light - just as Jesus baptized souls by immersing them in water - this has the same effect.

Pray for Peace. It is only through your prayers that we can intervene more fully to bring our whole planet into the Light. We pray along with you. We are part of you. We are one soul divided by the different strata of Earth, but all living the same life. Whatever happens to one, happens to us all, only on levels you just now comprehend.

It is Fall now on your surface, and all is dying for the Earth is gearing for her rebirth into Light. Just as the Fall changes to Winter, and Winter to Spring, your hearts are going through a rebirthing process that is carrying you speedily into the photon belt of Light. You will be ready for the merger and will rejoice at the impact when suddenly you find yourself illuminated and seeing the world around you through the eyes of God. It will be a speedy delivery into Light - and, yes, you will find us there, waiting for you as we always have.

World Trade Center Inner Planes Electoral Vote

Today the Earth is relatively quiet as humanity contemplates the events of the past week.

Although this was a heinous act and atrocity against mankind, it was not accidental. Those ones who chose to be there at that time had already chosen to leave the Earth and continue their ascension from the other side of the veil. They just left sooner than they normally would have - but not that much sooner. No one is caught in a catastrophe who has not chosen it on their subconscious level. Remember that there are no accidents - regardless of the magnitude of the incident - and this is no exception.

Now we will speak of the brother and sisterhood that prevail in the wake of this tragedy. This tragedy had welded people together - communities' all over the Earth - in an embrace of love and unity and brotherhood. It has closed the gap of separation between peoples, showing that you are all involved in the same struggle of life and death, and showing that you are all one in the face of calamity that you all share the same feelings and same hopes, and mainly that you all share the same prayers for your lost ones. This sameness is a big factor that has melded large groups of people together in a way that your past complacency could not.

We implore you to keep vigilant and to know beyond a doubt that the God you pray to hears every thought, every word, every gesture - and knows that the majority of people on Earth call for peace and justice in their hearts. And we mean justice neither vengeance nor retaliation - but justice heretofore not known in these past centuries.

These events of the past week have not hindered Earth's or humanity's ascension plan, but rather, have unified humanity to such an extent that in actuality the ascension has been furthered and heightened and quickened - although you who live in 3rd dimensional bodies cannot as yet fathom this. But soon you will see how this has enabled the ascension to go forth even more quickly, as the waves have snapped up even more and more people as a result of their abrupt awakening in the face of this immense tragedy and loss of lives.

Remember that God's Light never fails and that the Divine Plan for Earth is more intact than ever, and, more than ever, is now the time for all the Light workers to trust in the Divine Plan for the ascension of Earth and humanity. For the Light never gives up nor relinquishes its position. It may recede a bit, then comes back mightier in force and mightier in its resolve to move humanity up the scale of evolution to where these tragedies no longer can occur.

So you see, all is well on Earth and all is going according to Divine Plan. And what seems like a setback is really a speeding up of your ascension if you look deeper into the overall picture.

This has resulted in a vast awakening and a reversal that dark forces had not anticipated.

These terrorist tragedies do not fragment people. Rather, they unify them in their resolve to find peace on Earth. The hell that the darkness wants to promote lies inside those individuals who perpetrate these events, and as long as people do not buy into that reality of darkness, then peace and Heaven on Earth will prevail. Even though many millions of American people want revenge, no one wants war on American soil, and deep down in people's heart spaces, all cry for peace on Earth and justice to prevail. In fact, all humanity that is constructive to life - and this is the vast majority of people on Earth all want peace and love to prevail.

This is the call we all hear under the Earth and in the higher dimensions. The call for peace is so loud that it deafens everything else out. These calls are speeding up the ascension plan as nothing else could have, because when angry people call for revenge, they are exhibiting their hurts and scars from their past, but when interviewed on the Inner Planes at night, they all, with very few exceptions, choose peace.

So this is the vote we go by - the Inner Planes Electoral Vote - where all vote for peace without ballot tampering. It is the true vote and only vote that prevails. So rest assured that all is going according to Divine Will and that humanity will, indeed, ascend even sooner now.

You are the showcase of the Universe and you are surmounting and surpassing all obstacles being put in your way, and there will be more to come. For the dark is not done nor have they, as yet, given up. They will strike again, trying to thwart your passage into Light. But they will fail, as the resolve of the Light workers is too great and humanity is responding to the Light, not the dark.

Know that your world is safe. This drama will play itself out until there are only the "light" players left, as all the dark players will have vacated the premises and exited the stage. Their darkness will be gone and only the Light will prevail. Know that our hearts are filled with love for humanity, and as we watch the scenario from below, we feel your sadness and hear your calls for peace. We join our hearts with yours, magnifying your voices for peace on Earth.

Our foresight protects us underground, for we do not act without weighing the outcome of our actions or without seeing the possible future consequences. Some day you will have this foresight, this vision to see the future based on your choices before you make them. Always opt for peace and love, and your future will always bring it to you. What you choose is what you get.

So we down in the Hollow Earth give you our strength and stand with you in your resolve to bring all humanity into the Light so that we, as one planet united in the Love of God, can finally ascend as a whole and move on to our destiny of Galactic Unity and Galactic Ascension for the whole galaxy.

We Monitor the Milky Way Galaxy

Pay no heed to the outbursts of negativity and hostile warfare -

they are like a naughty child, just having an outburst that soon subsides into calmness and peace.

We in the Hollow Earth monitor your whole Earth. We have our amino-based computers that show us everything that is happening everywhere in our Galaxy and Universe and, of course, on Earth's surface. This is one of our "jobs," to keep track of everything simultaneously, and to plug the Confederation of Planets into the trouble spots on Earth as they occur.

Another war on Earth must not be tolerated. This is the end times - the end of war, the end of hate, negativity, anger, jealousy, competition, and fear.

Sleeping Giants of Yore

We speak to you from the fabled Library of Porthologos inside the Earth, but a step away from you in consciousness. You reach us by stepping down in your thoughts and, extending yourself and your imagination into our library, looking around, and "seeing" us. We stand there waiting for your entry.

Today we will talk about the Sleeping Giants from your folklore. These giants are Beings from the Hollow Earth who took residence on the surface thousands of years ago. In your folklore, you speak of them as sleeping for hundreds of years, and then awakening to find themselves in another time zone. Yes, they traveled from inside the Earth and lived on your surface for hundreds and thousands of years, studying humanity's surface population and then returning inside to report their findings. They did grow long beards, and many stories were written about them and their Herculean feats on the surface.

Know that Earth is populated with many different Beings from many different star systems, all here for the same purpose - to grow and evolve in consciousness, and to understand how humans evolve. The surface is a testing ground and experimenting station for growth and evolvement. The first four letters in "evolvement" are "love" spelled backwards. It is through love that you evolve. It is so simple - and yet it still eludes so many surface dwellers. Love is the glue - and it is through you, each and every one of you, that your world moves into higher states of consciousness, and it's all through love - love of yourself and love for your "other" selves. As you all come together in greater harmony and unity, you will feel yourselves and your reality shifting into higher vibrations of love and peacefulness, and you will gingerly step into the higher dimensions where you will begin to feel and see us. We are in these higher dimensions. For even as we reside "below" you, we are beside you. This is how "oneness" manifests.

Your world is rapidly changing and waking up, due in large part to the shock of the World Trade Center attack on September 11, 2001. This was a world emergency wake-up call, perpetrated by the dark forces in an attempt to wake you up to their presence. They have delved so deep into darkness that they have gone full circle and are now circling back into Light, and their terror is shocking people into their wake-up zone, affecting them in a polarity opposite of the dark's intention. The sleeping masses are finally being shocked into awakening to who they are - like the Sleeping Giants of yore.

You are all the Sleeping Giants who came to Earth's surface and fell into a great sleep - and who are finally awakening to what is being perpetrated on the surface. You've been caught in a great lie, believing everything the newspapers and media tell you, and never questioning the news source from whence it comes. Well, it all comes from the same one source - your government-controlled media - one viewpoint, theirs, which they program into your belief system.

As people awaken from their deep slumber of the ages, they begin to question and this is the awakening period. Soon you will all jump out of your beds and stand free with us in the higher realms of consciousness. Your Cetacean brothers and sisters wait for you there, too.

We have great monitors in the Library of Porthologos where we view surface conditions and follow your earthly lives. Nothing surprises us anymore, as we've seen it all, history repeating itself over and over again. But now we see something different - through the repetition of events - we see humanity waking up and remembering that there's more than war and strife and struggle and lack and limitation. They are remembering the Divine within them and this remembrance is the awakening.

Once a critical mass of people is awakened, you will all float into higher consciousness instantly and the past will be a dream. We wait for you at the gates of your consciousness, and as the floodgates open, the waves of Light will carry you through. As Light workers, you have all prepared for this for eons, and now it is here.

The European Euro

We transmit to you directly from the Library of Porthologos, where many of us spend most of our time. Although our time frame differs from yours, we still tell time and arrange our schedules and days.

The Hollow Earth is rejoicing at the magnitude of the rise in Earth's consciousness as witnessed by the announcement of the Euro on today's news, bringing many European countries together as ONE. This is a great step for the surface population, leading to a United Earth World.

We in the Hollow Earth have one system for all of us, which keeps us unified in all areas of commerce and life. It is a big step taken, and many more countries will follow.

Confusion and Turmoil on the Surface

Your health is linked to your wealth. By this we mean your emotional health - your feeling body - for the healthier you "feel," the clearer and purer your thoughts and feelings, the clearer your intentions will be. It is your intent that goes out into the Universal Fields of Light, and brings you back what you send out for. Every thought is a call, and every call has an answer.

So attune yourselves to your thoughts and your feelings, and monitor what you are sending out. If you send out only what is positive, that is what you will receive.

This is a time of great confusion and turmoil on the surface, as people are being awakened by the string of events unfolding. Stay within your own center, go deep down, and feel only the calmness and tranquility that exists within you, and radiate this out to counteract the negativity and upheaval that is going on around you. This is your purpose; this is what it means to "Hold the Light." It means you are holding the Light that ever exists within you, and choosing to reflect only the light, and not the confusion around you. So go within, and stay within, even as you are existing in all outward appearances. It is so simple, yet so profound.

In the Hollow Earth, we all live from our heart center and radiate only the tranquility within us. This tranquility permeates the whole cavity of the Earth and brings us the health and riches that surround us always. As surface folk begin to live from within their heart center, this purity and strength and peacefulness will permeate your physical bodies and surface conditions, and gently bring you the peace that abides within us and inside our Earth.

Peace Is The Answer

We bring you tidings from the Hollow Earth located in the innermost cavity of your planet.

We dwell here in peace and prosperity and great abundance. We wear precious gems and gold that adorn our bodies and homes, and everyone has as many as they could ever want. Everything is in prolific abundance - including peace and unconditional love. For it is this peace and love that creates abundance and prosperity and longevity of life. This is the secret - the magic to life.

Just live in peace and harmony and love with one another, and heaven on Earth is yours. It is truly magic. For peaceful living can only bring more peace and great riches beyond your 3rd dimensional imagination. Peace is the answer to all your societal ills. Love is the answer to all your family and relationship problems. Peace is the answer to your economic woes and stock market fluctuations. Peaceful co-existing is the purpose of life and the reason you are here.

Don't let it elude you, and don't let 9/11 and other tragedies detract you from feeling peace within yourself. These events are but ploys to detract you from the peace that already exists within each of you. These events are purposely orchestrated to push humanity off the course of your impending ascension. No matter what transpires on your surface world, stay calm and centered within your soul and "feel peace". It is only through the feelings that peacefulness can emerge. Hold this peacefulness and let it extend out onto your surface, and touch every soul you come in contact with. This is how you spread peace and counteract the darkness around your Earth.

The Forces of Light are here in great numbers surrounding your Earth and every man, woman and child. Our Central Sun has sent Legions of Angels to guide and protect you, as the energies coming to Earth are so powerful now that everything not of Love is being pushed to the surface for healing.

We in the Hollow Earth are insulated from the chaos above, for the Earth is a great insulator and provides a protective shield all around us. We can be in contact with you, but cannot be contacted by negativity. It just can't reach us. Our shield of protection is just too strong. We've woven a force field around us that is impenetrable to everything that is not of the Light. We are secure and safe inside the Earth for it is the only way we can exist and evolve.

When you achieve these peaceful living conditions, we can then emerge and welcome you into the Confederation of Planets, where you will be shown how to change your world back into Paradise.

Our Immortality

We have waited all day in joy, knowing that we would make

our connection today, at the end of your day. We are joyous to be here with you today, partnering with you to bring our messages to our brothers and sisters above ground. Thank you for keeping your appointment with us.

Today we will speak about time and how fleeting it is on the surface. You count your days, your minutes, your seconds, and register them all in your bodies, thinking that aging signifies the passage of time. As people age, time passes. As buildings deteriorate, time passes. This is time on the surface, and it is all an illusion. Time really does not exist - it can't exist - and we are a prime example. Our bodies don't age and our buildings don't deteriorate. So does this mean that there's no time in the Inner Earth, but only time on the surface? You would think so, wouldn't you? But our lives attest to the fact that through your passage of time, our bodies stay young, no matter how much time passes on the surface. You measure your time with aging, but we don't age. Does this mean 'time stands still' for us? Or does it rather mean that you're using an inappropriate measurement?

Your bodies wouldn't age if you didn't count the days and years as 'getting older'. If you counted the days and years as your journeys around the sun, instead of 'aging', then 30 years would mean 30 trips around the sun, instead of 30 years 'old'. 'Trips' don't age you, but 'years old' does. If you just change the words from 'years old' to 'trips', you gain your immortality. It's all in your beliefs and your speech. Your speech and your thoughts make it so.

In the Hollow Earth we know there's no such thing as aging, because we never see it. We know there's no such thing as time as you experience it because here everything is in a perpetual state of 'youthfulness' and 'newness'. Everything looks as new as the day it was created, including our bodies. We exist in a state of divine perfection, in an environment of 'timelessness'.

We never 'hurry' and are never 'late', and we never 'kill time' as you do on the surface. Have you noticed how this is a favorite saying of yours? It's as if time were your enemy, and whenever you have some extra time you 'kill it' . You are in a rush to use up all the time in your life, so that the end comes fast, and you don't have to 'feel'. You just stay busy, watch the years of your life pass, and hope it ends without leaving any 'extra' time on your hands. For what would you do with 'extra' time? The thought would scare you, for it would leave you time to feel yourself, to feel your life, and feeling is what everyone wants to avoid. So without enough time left at the end of each day, you can avoid 'feeling' and just continue a robot-like existence.

You can stop time. Just start feeling yourself in every moment and prolong this feeling, this consciousness of yourself. You can actually expand your 'time', and prolong your youthfulness, by not getting caught up in 'time'. If it starts slipping away from you, you can stop to recapture it by feeling yourself deeply in the moment. It's all about awareness. If you lose yourself in your day you lose a segment of your life. If you're aware of yourself throughout your day, you gain immortality; for you're focusing on the 'now'.

You would love our easy life style and slow, harmonious ways. We have 'time' to think things out, to talk things out, before we make choices. We're never forced to choose because 'time is running out' or there's a 'deadline'. These are obstacles that you've created on the surface, and they just don't exist 'down here'.

We Have The Eyes Of Falcons

Today it is bright and glorious inside the Hollow Earth, as our Inner Sun is always shining and there are never any clouds in our sky. Our vision is always clear, and we can see for miles around our inner cities, and across our sky to the other side of our Inner Earth. We have the eyes of falcons, with intense, precise vision. No one here wears glasses, as our sight is perfect. Seeing is believing, and soon you will be able to see us with your inner vision, and wonder how you had never seen us before. As your consciousness climbs in frequency, so does the perfection of your body expand to every cell and organ, until you return to the divine perfection that you are.

Our Oceans and Beaches

Good morning. It is Mikos calling to you from the ocean shore in the Hollow Earth, where I am walking along the beach watching the waves lap the sand. Our oceans are large, nay huge in comparison to yours, with waves larger in size and stronger in force. The oceans flow swiftly around our Inner Globe, and ebb and flow in tides affected by the Earth's outer moon just as your tides are. For the magnetic pull of the moon is felt inside the Earth as well.

We all spend much of our time on the beaches, walking on the sand along the shore, and swimming in the ocean's clean, clear water. The water in our oceans and rivers is composed of living consciousness, and it is our water's consciousness that keeps us young forever.

Your water is the elixir of life, and in its pure state, it can change your bodies and actually bring the dead back to life. It can bring the life force back into each and every cell, thereby increasing the flow of consciousness in your whole body and bringing full consciousness back into every living cell. This quickening can move you beyond all earthly sicknesses and diseases, and give you the physical perfection and physical immortality you all yearn for. So drink your water 'consciously', and know that soon our pure water will arrive on the surface to cure all the ills of your people and bring them back into a higher state of consciousness.

There are already some bodies of water on the surface that are known for their curative effects, and people by the millions go to them. Soon all your bodies of water will have these curative effects and more, as we prepare ourselves to emerge from below ground and merge with you on the surface. Your bodies yearn to be freed from the distortion of sickness and disease, and yearn to feel the illumination of God's Light from within. Our water will dissolve all negativity and blockages and bacteria, so that your cells are clear to radiate the Light from God that is always flowing through you.

Your Inner Heart's Flame is always ablaze with God's Light, but the current density of the cells quench the Light's illuminating effect and instead of the Light blazing forth like a golden sun, its rays become splintered and distorted and stuck. Water and Light are necessary for life, and your cells need to be purified to hold the great Light that is emanating from your Heart's Flame, which is a true and actual flame that is lit inside your heart and composed of the consciousness of the Creator flowing through you.

So know that as the pollution of the surface has intensified, so has the pollution inside your body. Whatever you do to the planet, you do to yourself. If you as a species stop polluting your earth, water and air, you will stop polluting your bodies.

They are inextricably connected, as you can see. But this can all be reversed, as you can also see, and we will reverse all these conditions that are against life, when we come to the surface in the not too distant future.

Our Water Talks

Our shorelines are packed with the purest of sand, white colored and soft and crystal clear specs of the smoothest particles you have ever stepped on. Walking on our sandy beaches is akin to having the best foot massage possible. And we do walk on our beaches for this very purpose, for its massage soothes our feet and mind simultaneously. Our ocean's waves lap our shorelines with the purest and cleanest of water you have ever seen or tasted. And the temperature is always perfect for our bodies. Not too warm and not too cold. We walk into our oceans where it is shallow, and swim out great distances without ever getting tired or cold. No one here ever drowns. This is unheard of and unimaginable. We are all great swimmers, and our oceans and lakes support us so that we stay on top of the water.

Our water has consciousness, and talks to us while we are immersed in it. Yes, our water talks. When we swim, our water becomes part of our body, and we are one body, one ocean, swimming along the currents and through the waves. We merge ourselves completely with the water's consciousness and our swim is a trip in consciousness itself. It is so much more than what you experience in your surface lakes and oceans, where the consciousness of your water has become so densified and polluted that it has lost its voice and vitality and life force.

It weakly calls out to you, but you don't hear it. It calls out to you for help. It calls out to you to stop polluting it, to stop bombarding it with ELF sound waves, to stop the whaling ships and underwater experiments, and oil spills, and submarines, and cruise ships from destroying and poisoning its life force. But alas, it rests on deaf ears. For the children of Earth are still deaf to the destruction they are causing the Earth. It's only the greedy politicians who know what they are doing, and they do it purposely to destroy the Earth for their own personal gain, in the name of bolstering the economy. Everything is for the economy, and nothing for the Earth or its people. Families don't count anymore, only the state of the economy counts. You never hear about the 'state of the family' on the news, it's always the 'state of the economy' you hear about. Well, when there's no longer any families alive, there won't be an economy either.

So help yourself by helping your Earth. It's only through your returning your surface oceans and lands to their pristine state that you will return to a perfect economy where everyone lives in abundance and perfect health.

Our Inner Earth Oceans are Sanctuaries to all Marine Life

The Inner Earth's Oceans contain all of the life that's in the upper oceans and more. Our oceans are teeming with life, and all of the marine forms live in harmony with one another.

All are on a vegetarian diet and do not hunt others. All live in harmony. All the marine life is very evolved compared to the life in the surface oceans. All are used to the peace and safety of our waters, and all are accessible to us. We all communicate directly to the Cetaceans and fish, and live cooperatively and in peace with one another.

Since we are all on a vegetarian diet, we don't hunt the Whales, go fishing or farm shrimp.

Therefore, Mother Nature is free to evolve in our oceans and our oceans are sanctuaries to all ocean life. We just call to whomever we want to talk to, and they swim to our shores and converse with us. It would seem truly magical to you, but to us it is commonplace. Remember, all of us in the Hollow Earth know we are ONE.

There are numerous underwater caverns, where we go 'scuba' diving and explore the intricacies and complexities of life beneath the oceans. There are so many different kinds of organisms and plants and corals that are hidden in the ocean caverns that are beauteous to see. We love to dive and swim, explore and commune with the nature elementals in the oceans. There's a whole other civilization beneath our seas that we live in peace and cooperative partnership with. How wonderful to exist in a climate of peaceful exchange that we have forged beneath the Earth.

Your surface whales and dolphins sometimes swim through the underground ocean tunnels to visit and commune with us. They stay a short while and then return to the surface. They wish they could stay longer, but know their mission is above ground, and hesitatingly leave for the great swim upwards.

Food and Elements of Nature

Greetings from the Hollow Earth! Today we will talk about our Earth, our dear planet that gives all life a home to evolve on. Know that your home is also the home of countless other species that depend upon it for shelter, food and a place to live.

Your corporations act as if the land belongs to them alone, with no regard for other life forms. Space on Earth is designated for all species to share equally, for all are here to evolve their souls and all are here to enjoy their life spans. As this is especially true for humans, all other species have come to help and bolster the life of humans by giving them oxygen, food and clothing. All you have is being given to you as gifts from other species. The trees give you oxygen, the animals give you clothing, and the crops give you food. All of these are live, conscious beings, here in service to Earth and to all life forms. Trees, animals, crops, plants, Cetaceans and all ocean life, all need their habitats kept intact in order for them to survive and evolve, just as humans need their homes to live in to carry on their lives.

It is a travesty to destroy the natural habitats of other living beings just to pave more roads, make more shopping centers and erect more suburban tract homes. By cutting down trees and moving animals out of their homes, you destroy their lives, thereby endangering yours.

For in order for all life to evolve, there must be an ecological balance on Earth. Humans have destroyed this delicate ecological balance, thinking only of themselves and not honoring the right of other life forms to claim their inheritance and their share of land and resources on Earth. This pushing off, and moving out, of other species is causing a severe imbalance to the Earth, which is leading to the devastation of flora and fauna, and ultimately to the destruction of all life everywhere.

For all life is interdependent and intricately interconnected. What happens to one happens to all; and mankind is now waking up and starting to realize this interconnectedness.

We, here in the Hollow Earth, have learned this many eons ago, and base our life on this connection to all life everywhere. This is also your connection to God. For once you realize your connection to all life, you automatically are reconnected to God, the Source of All That Is.

And it is this connection that will evolve your soul and move you into your ascension. When all mankind awake to their connection to all other life, they suddenly find themselves connected to God and their trip home begins.

We have already made this trip, and find ourselves secure in the 'Garden of Eden' inside Earth. Paradise is the destination of your trip too, and many are now living lives of joy and abundance right here on the surface of Earth. You really don't have to go anywhere to enjoy your life fully. You just have to make your 'connection in' and everything you ever dreamed of will come to you effortlessly. For this is the way life was intended to be.

Here in the Hollow Earth, we watch and pray and send our Love to you daily. We encourage you to connect in consciousness with us, for through your connection we can send you our energy to energize your body and feed your spirit.

Food Takes on the Mass Consciousness of the Community It's Grown In

You, on the surface, live in misery, lack, and trepidation, because you have separated yourself from God, thinking that you know best, or more than the Creator. Your lives have been blessed with the riches and abundance of the Earth, and yet you turn away from Her, in your disdain, using your own methods of farming instead of Natures'. Mother Earth has always produced an abundance of crops for all who work with her, using Nature's Law of Rotation and Nature's Law of turning the soil into itself and letting it lie fallow to recover and restore its nutrients. By continual planting of the same crops over and over, dosed with toxic fertilizers and chemicals, you kill the rich nutrients of the Earth, leaving crops that are devoid of nutrition and devoid of the Life Force.

People of old always worked with the Devas, the Guardians of the soil; and by working together, and allowing the Earth herself to manage and make decisions for the growth of crops that are planted, the yields were always large nay, enormous and brimming with the force of life pulsing through each atom. It is this force of life in each atom and cell, this pulsation, this quickening, which is the Immortal Elixir of life. It is the secret of staying "young" forever.

The Devas are returning to Earth after a long absence and are quietly helping those few people who are turning to them, to rebuild the soil with life enriching nutrients that will nourish and sustain the cells in our human bodies. The Devas are glorious beings who want to work with all humans, whether you farm or not, or just garden. They want to return to a partnership with you, so that all people can learn the magic of the soil, the magic of planting and harvesting again, the magic of growing your own food, in your own locality, for your own consumption. Food shipped to you from other localities from far away states, does not vibrate with your local surroundings or your own particular pulse of life.

Everything is a reflection of your immediate surroundings, including your auras that surround you; and everything you touch or are near picks up your pulsating atoms, and these atoms become part of the soil and part of the vibration of everything you grow. So don't you think that you would be healthier to absorb only those vibrating atoms in your food that originate from your own self and from the community you vibrate with, rather than from an unknown locality that you are out of synchronicity with? There is so much to think of here, and much to understand about the nature of life, and how we all adapt to the particular locality we live in and how we become that locality. We are the environment that we live in, just as much as the crops we grow are.

It is confusing to your body cells to be ingesting foods from out of your immediate locale because they do not resonate with your lifestyles, your thoughts, or your feelings. Instead, you imbibe, you actually "eat" other people's thoughts and feelings and they become yours not knowing the danger and incompatibility this has on your digestive system and overall operation of all your organs, all your growth hormones, all your glands, and everything that makes you "you." Your ingesting of the thoughts of other people results in fears and phobias that aren't even your own, and then you wonder where this all came from.

Know that in order to have healthy and strong bodies, you need to feed them with only foods from your own local communities. This will enhance your life force and bring balance to your thoughts and feelings, because you will be reinforcing and strengthening your desires and dreams — which comprise the mass consciousness of a community.

This is why your world is out of sync, because it is out of sync with nature. Call on the Devas, ask them all to return, tell them you want to learn from them and work in tandem with them, to restore life to the soil and life to your bodies. Without this life force, your bodies decay and wither, and although your cells were meant to stay young and never age, they lack the life force to sustain themselves.

Your current civilization has moved further and further away from the soil, the trees, and the animals, into the ivy tower of technology, with no windows to look outside at their surroundings. They have closed the door to communing with nature, and wonder why they feel so alone and so needy, no matter how much money they have.

We implore you. Earth people, to return to Nature. She beckons you back to be one with her again, and to follow in the footsteps of your ancestors, the Native American Indians, who knew the land as part of themselves, who lived with nature, and honored and revered her bounty, and who learned from her, always using her own way to grow crops, and never forcing her to work against herself.

Spend time outdoors, not locked up in your houses. Spend time just sitting with the trees and walking in the woods, and notice the life force returning to you, invigorating you and balancing your emotional body. Nature is a great antidote for your society's ills and if s free for all to receive. You don't need to consult a physician for a prescription; the trees will dispense it to you for free. Why do you think they are here only to grace your landscape?

The trees are Majestic Beings, evolved beyond anything your thoughts can picture. And they wait for you to recognize them also as the stewards of the land, as the Cetaceans are the stewards of the sea, always giving you the oxygen you need, and absorbing the pollutants you create. And what do you do in return for this gift of life? You cut them down, you move them out of your way, and you ignore them. They are yearning to communicate with you, yearning to feel your touch and embrace you in their love and energy. Go to them, talk to them, sit with them, as they stand vigilant over your homes and communities as protectors of your very lives. Talk to them, and they will answer. They have been waiting eons to have humans reconnect to them again.

Nature will free you. You will regain your balance, you will regain your will to dream and to rebuild your lives in accordance with the Laws of Nature, not the laws of man. We, here in the Hollow Earth, are one with nature, one with all life, and one with God. This is why we live such long lives and are so healthy. We know we are all a part of our planet. and our planet is a part of us. When we work with nature, we work as one. When we ignore nature, we ignore ourselves. This is a Universal Law that is crucial to your survival as a species.

We bring your attention to this, so you can protect your planet so that you have a home to evolve on. Since you can't evolve in space, we wonder why you so blatantly destroy your home?

You would marvel at the wonders in the Inner Earth, the wonders of beauty and the "down to earth" sensible lifestyles we have, all because we apply the Universal Law of the Oneness of all life. I bid you good day.

Our Fields of Grains

Our fields of grains sparkle and thrive and are perfectly touched by the "sun" and rain to produce the most luscious of crops that are so pleasing to our palates and so invigorating for our bodies. Our food pulses with the force of life, and when eaten by us transfers the life force into our very cells, which results in perfect health and longevity of years.

This is the secret of life; this is the hidden fountain of youth you've all been looking for on your surface. It is found in the Earth herself, just waiting to give you its life force if you will but follow nature's laws of planting and harvesting crops, using only nature herself to direct the process and oversee the growth. With the great forces of nature working with you, you don't need to add anything to the soil, and the harvests are always magnificent in size and nutrients and taste.

This strength given us by our foods enables us to perform Herculean feats with our bodies that you would consider impossible. We can walk and run extremely long distances without tiring, and swim for hours at a time. We are not tired at the end of a day's "work", because nothing we do is "work". It is all joy and ease, and contentment is felt at the end of each day.

Our lives are truly wonderful, and we have much to feel blessed for. But we have created this Utopia ourselves, and so can, and so will, you. For your future is to be glorious. You are about to break through this density into heaven. And this heaven is right here on Earth.

Right now only half of the planet resides here, but soon the whole planet will be in the heaven you've been searching for. For heaven is not in another place; its location is right here on Earth. Right here where you live. You only have to bring it here through your higher consciousness. For heaven is just a frequency, and you are now rising rapidly toward accessing that frequency. And We, here in the Hollow Earth, are applauding your desire and determination to grow in awareness and reach the frequency of ascension that is plummeting to Earth from the Great Central Sun. Your Father/ Mother, God and Goddess, Alpha and Omega, are bringing you home, back into their bosoms of love, where We will all dwell for the rest of eternity.

Our Environment and Water

We feel the climate changes from above, just as you do, even though we are physically removed from them and nestled snugly inside the Hollow Earth. For we track the weather conditions and anomalies on the surface and can tell when a cataclysm (earth quake, hurricane, etc.) is about to occur. We are meteorologists too, and specialize in monitoring the weather conditions on the surface. This way, we can tell where pockets of darkness and negative thought forms that create weather imbalances are coming from. We then focus our love light on these areas to disperse and dematerialize them. This is one of the many contributions we render to the surface.

If surface folk knew the importance of keeping their mental and feeling bodies balanced, they could change the world overnight from one of chaos to one of peace. It's all in the balance. As each of you brings balance to your life, the Earth gains that measure and it goes out to all life, which in turn adds this amount of balance to their lives. . .and so it goes. It means to monitor and control your thoughts and feelings, just as you would monitor and control a science experiment in a lab to produce the desired results.

Well, think of your life as an experiment, and you being given the experience of learning to control all aspects of yourself. This is the key to a harmonious life and to peace on Earth. Each person plays such an integral role in bringing peace, that you would be amazed if you could 'actually see' how your thoughts and feelings go out into the world and touch others. It is a Law of Life that whatever you think and feel creates your reality and affects others as well - including all the other Kingdoms on Earth.

You are powerful, aren't you? Now harness your power into constructive building blocks that will bring peace to everyone around you and that will promote peace on Earth. It all starts with you, each individual on Earth. Take control of your life, and you can control the weather and receive the benefit of warm, sunshiny days, with gentle breezes that caress your skin. This is the 'true' weather control system, and we've installed it in the Hollow Earth. And you can install it for free on the surface, with 'no' installation fees.

Not only can you balance the weather using this technique, but you can balance your body and free it from stress and the unbalancing factors that cause disease. All these with no charge either. Everything you wish for, you can create from within yourself for free, and freely dispense it to others and to Mother Earth herself - thus healing all life everywhere. What a gift you have stored within you, and you can dispense your healing without ever spending thousands of dollars going to medical school; for you have already graduated. You're here on Earth to practice what you already know, and the knowledge is stored in the memory banks of your cells.

We always go within to our inner storehouse, to access all we need to live lives of peace and abundance. God's Light within us never fails. It is only your failure to go within to find the inner storehouse that keeps piling up for your use. By now, you have quite an oversupply just waiting for you to tap into and start bringing it into your outer lives.

Oceans and Mountains in the Hollow Earth

The Earth's Interior is the mirror image of the surface foundation. Everything is in reverse order in the inside of the Earth. The mountain ranges are in direct proportion to the dimensions of the Earth's cavity, and tower above the landscape. The oceans are larger than life, and flow calmly and swiftly around the inside of the globe. The air is crisp and clean, and the sand is white. The Central Sun is dimmer than the sun on the outside, and reflects the Light from the Heavens.

The cities are all nestled in lush woodlands, overflowing with flowers and huge trees. There is green growth surrounding all man-made structures. Everything is in perpetual blossom and bloom. It is a land of wonder and beauty.

All is in perfect proportion to the size of the circumference of the interior. Everything is larger than life even the great Beings who inhabit the interior are larger than the mortals on the outside. All is beauty, and all is in a heavenly state of bliss.

Just picture the interior foundation reflecting the exterior foundation; with mountain ranges higher, and the ocean currents swifter, and the green land growth lush beyond compare. You do not need to picture a change in the contour of the land. It is still in its pristine beauty, and replicates how life on the surface once was. The exact location of the mountain ranges and oceans is not necessary to know at this time. What is necessary to know is that this Inner World exists, and co-exists with the surface, under peaceful and contrary conditions.

Weather, Tunnels and Spaceports in the Hollow Earth.

Know that cataclysmic weather conditions are in store for your surface population. Many negative thought forms are being released from your bodies and from the Earth, and these are causing drastic atmospheric imbalances, resulting in tornadoes, earthquakes, and other variable conditions.

Up north, where it's colder and the days are shorter, people will begin to see a change in their weather and seasonal patterns. The days will grow longer and the seasons will begin to merge into one another, just as they do in the Hollow Earth. In the Hollow Earth, there is a constant temperature in the low 70's. This "constant" temperature allows the people to live in relative ease and comfort, for no obstacles impede their activities.

The Hollow Earth is a Paradise, with tall, graceful mountains jutting into the "sky"; and large, clear, clean lakes and oceans that abound with life. The diet in the Hollow Earth is strictly vegetarian, and people are healthy, robust, and strong. They, too, have isolated themselves from the surface population, although they come and leave the Earth freely using the spacecraft that are kept there in the Spaceport in the inside of the Earth. So although they are inside the Earth, they have freedom and health, and abundance and peace all the necessary components of life that you on the surface have been crying out for.

There is free travel between the subterranean cities and the Hollow Earth through the tunnels, using our electromagnetic trains that can take us from one part of the Earth to another in a fraction of the time it takes you on the surface. Our transportation is quick and efficient, and bums no fuels. Therefore, there's no pollution underground.

We long for the day when you on the surface can travel freely to the Hollow Earth, where you'll he greeted with great joy and love. It is this return, to the Land of Eden, that you are all crying out for. We, too, await this day, as all of us in the subterranean cities, will join with you in the celebration, merging all our civilizations into One.

UNDERGROUND TUNNEL SYSTEM

There are tunnels intertwining throughout the planet, connecting every large city or state. The Inner Earth inhabitants can reach most of their destinations within hours, if not minutes. This underground network of passageways has been used for eons. They are more connected below than we are above. They can travel anywhere freely without making reservations, paying large sums of money or spending days at airports, train stations, or in cars.

Our Homes

Our library rooms are all environmentally harmonious with our outdoor surroundings, and all are open to the green of our outdoors and rich fragrances of our flowers. Our rooftops are open as well, as there are none. There is nothing above us to separate us from heaven. Our oiffice room space is exposed to all the elements, and all the Hollow Earth elements harmoniously and joyously intermingle and interact in a state of divine perfection. So we don't need rooftops to protect ourselves from them, as they work directly with us - not against us. And because all our buildings are round, we never have to dust, because dust never accumulates.

We live dust free lives in our circular buildings and homes. Geometric shapes have certain properties, and in a circle the energy freely moves and revolves, carrying dust particles along with it so that the dust never settles in corners - since a corner does not exist in a circle. So as a dust particle moves into a room, the energy flow also carries it out. It is more efficient than a vacuum cleaner, because a storage bag isn't necessary. Soon this architectural principle will be prevalent on Earth and all your structures will be circular in shape.

Jewels, Diamonds, and Crystals

We reside here, in the Hollow Earth, amongst great richness, and live in great palaces infused with Light. To you, it would seem as a f antasyland, but to us it is real, as we created it from our own God Selves. We created homes for Gods and Goddesses, and this is where we dwell.

We dwell amongst richness your eyes cannot yet conceive of. Every possible convenience is at our fingertips and our environment is more beautiful than you can imagine. Our homes are set in the lushness of the countryside that abounds all around us, and are built right into the natural environment, surrounded by lakes and streams.

We have no cities like yours. We have only "country" that never ceases to amaze even Us. The trees and flowers are vibrant with pulsating hues and shapes, and caress our homes and land. Everything is "monumental", as you would term it. Even our trees and mountains are double the height of yours, and of course our bodies are taller and larger in frame. The width and girth of our figures more than doubles yours, and our fruits and vegetables are huge in comparison to yours. All our foods are organic, as we are in tune with Mother Earth, and she personally directs their growth.

We live in grand palaces made of crystallized stones that are embedded with jewels from the Earth. These crystallized stones create a magnetic field and radiance that nurtures and balances our bodies and fills us with the Life Force emanating from the Great Central Sun of our Universe. All things in our homes radiate the purity of God, and tune us to God's vibrations. For it is God's love that fills our homes and God's love that creates the richness in our lives.

Our homes are round and translucent, and blend into the countryside. By outward appearances they give us total privacy. But once within, we can see out in all directions around us.

This gives us a spacious feeling of vision, rather than being "locked in", as you are on the surface. Not only can we see out of our homes, but we can see out beyond the Earth, to the Stars in the sky. Our vision has no boundaries or barriers, wherever we are in the Hollow Earth. Our eyes and senses are free to roam the Universe, while our bodies remain inside the globe.

We Live Inside Caverns

Now that you are familiar with the Hollow Earth, we can "dig" further into your credibility and introduce another factor of our living arrangements underground. Underground, we do not live out in the open spaces the way you do on the surface. Our Hollow Earth cavity is pristine because we don't tread upon her inner surface nor build upon her. We don't have shopping malls and expanses of highways nor towering buildings. We live inside caverns, with openings facing inward toward the open, wide spaces of the Hollow cavity inside the Earth. Sure, we travel inside the cavity on our electromagnetic vehicles that levitate a few inches above the ground - but never touch the ground. We walk softly on the earthen paths and run along the streams, rivers and oceans, and climb the towering mountains. But that is the extent of our foot contact with the terrain. The rest we leave to nature's devas and elementals, as it is their land, too.

All our living activity takes place within our inner caverns, which are vast and wide and high and composed of crystalline rocks and gemstones and crystal arches radiating full-spectrum colored rainbows of sparkling light into our cavern atmosphere. Our walls are lined with natural rainbow-hued waterfalls, humidifying the air with the vibrancy and song of its water cascading down. Yes, our water sings - and its chorus brings our body cells into harmony, so that our bodies are always vibrating to our water and crystalline surroundings that keep us energized and vibrant all day long. We need little sleep because our cells are always tuned and in harmony to the natural rhythm of Mother Earth herself. When you are tuned like a tuning fork, then you carry the full life force of our Mother, and your battery never runs down.

Hence, there is little need for the long hours of sleep such as you experience it. You are drained and run-down after a day in your "sweatshops," but we are always as vibrant at the end of our days as we are when we begin them. We live "in" and "with" the Earth, whereas you live "outside" and "separate" from her. Hence, you are "cut off," while we are a "part" of her. This is the big difference.

Humanity was not meant to live on the Earth's rooftop, but inside her interior terrain. This was a big experiment that, unfortunately, backfired and resulted in alienation and "deep" separation from her life-giving body. Soon this will all be changed and remedied, and people will be living inside her, not on top of her. You live inside your house, not on its rooftop, don't you? Well, the same analogy applies to the Earth. There are vast caverns throughout the interior of the Earth, many already inhabited by many different kinds of beings who have been living unobtrusively in them for millennia.

Your Spiritual Hierarchy has been preparing housing for you inside these vast, uninhabited caverns in Earth's interior, and when it's time, you will all be moved en masse into them to continue your present incarnation inside Earth, not "on" her. You will encounter a "whole" new way of living that is wholesome and rich and perfect in every way. It will expand your consciousness and expand your horizon, and your horizon will be an inner horizon vaster than when you walk outdoors on the surface. A whole new horizon is waiting for you to experience.

Events will start happening fast now, as time is speeding up even faster as world karma is playing itself out. Just ride with the tide and know you are safe wherever you are. You are all being directed and guided from within, and you are all being provided for. What you witness through your media is only a "play," a drama that they want you to believe is real, just because the actors are real. But the actors are just "playing out their part" in the world's drama, and this is the biggest "hit" yet of the new millennium, playing on your TV and movie theater screens everywhere. Just turn the knob off, go within yourself, and feel and focus on world peace. Peace is the real movie, and the only "reel" to watch. Soon, you will see us, and soon you, too, will be living perfectly suited to your new way of life.

Inner Earth Caverns

Greetings from Earth's caverns! I am speaking to you today from my cavern inside the interior crust of the Hollow Earth.

Yes, there are caverns inside the Hollow Earth just as there are under the surface. The Earth is filled with caverns; everywhere you go on the planet there are caverns of such multitude and magnitude that the entire surface population can be comfortably housed inside.

In fact, this is how it is on all other planets in your solar system and beyond. The occupants all reside in inner domiciles, protected from the winds and sun of their solar system. This, indeed, will be the next step for humanity - to take residence inside the Earth herself for protection from the elements and forces of Nature that are bearing down on you from the outer atmospheric shell of Earth, and wreaking havoc on your cities in the form of hurricanes, tornados, earthquakes, winds, severe heat and cold extremes in temperature. The Earth is in the process of ridding herself of all pollution and may go through drastic measures to do so. This cleansing of her surface will also give those the opportunity to leave the Earth plane early and to continue their learning in the newly established temples and universities on the Inner Plane.

The hardships will enable those who stay to more quickly wake up to Earth's call and work with her and not against her. It will be a great opportunity for soul growth on Earth, and rare lessons will be available.

The caverns inside the Earth have been readied to accommodate the Earth's surface population, and they will all be brought inside when the time comes.

There's a web of tunnels crisscrossing throughout (or rather "through-in") the Earth's interior that will connect all caverns by electromagnetic vehicles that levitate and do not ever touch the ground as they whisk you through them from location to location. All is lit up in a soft iridescent glow, illuminating everything clearly while radiating a feeling of warmth inside the tunnel passageways.

The caverns will mirror your surface, except, of course, for the oceans, which you will have to travel into the Hollow Earth to access. The Hollow Earth is not that far away from the inner caverns - just minutes by electromagnetic vehicles, and they're all free. There's no transportation costs inside the Earth. In fact, there's no money at all. All is on a barter system and transportation is always free to all. You will be able to travel at will and finally explore the depths of the Earth as you begin to experience the depths of your own Being simultaneously. You, who choose to stay, are in for a great adventure in love and light and will witness the expansion of your universe from here on Earth.

DNA and Inner Doors of Consciousness

All people on Earth are from the same DNA blueprint, but evolution has created different outward appearances. So your appearance is determined dependent upon your location. These are not differences, just variations of body appearance. For within the body, lies the soul; and the souls of all humans come from the Divine Creator of All - are indeed a part of the Divine Creator - just embellished with Earthly characteristics and Earthly experiences that become different and distinct over eons of time. So what you see in others, is their Earthly sojourn, so to speak, and not their heavenly garment. This has confused humans for millennia, and resulted in separation and wars, instead of unity and peace.

We admonish you to look through God's eyes when you look at others, and see only God standing in the midst of you. You will see how rapidly your world conditions would change, if all would only look through God's eyes, always, which really are the eyes you look through when cleared of Earthly density and fear.

Take long walks through the countryside and breathe in the fragrant green-filled air. For the green of the countryside pulsates with the healing atoms that you all need so desperately to recover from the chaos of the city and your workplaces. For your city life depletes your life force, which the Trees and Nature can restore. The Trees are eager to help you, eager to give you their life-breathing oxygen that your city life consumes as rapidly as the Trees produce it. So rapidly, that now there is a great oxygen deficit on your surface and you all are feeling the effects of being oxygen-starved, due to your commerce and way of life.

We in the Hollow Earth are out in Nature 24 hours a day, as this is our only way of life. This is how we live because our surroundings are totally nature-made. We have no pollution producing cities. We have no asphalt or concrete suffocating Mother Earth's body. We have only trees and shrubs and grass and flowers everywhere we look. We have an abundance of pure oxygen, which renews and rebuilds our bodies 24 hours a day, resulting in our great strength and great energy levels, and clear thinking.

We wait for the time when you will be allowed to come 'down' and visit us, and witness for yourself our divine living conditions - which you can also create on the surface. Don't despair, for all in heaven are here to help you bring this heavenly way of existence down to Earth, so that all surface dwellers will at last experience the beauty and joy that was originally intended at the outset of this grand experiment on

Earth, over 14 million years ago.

Feel Your Heart As It Beats.

'Feel your heart as it beats.

Listen to your pulse as it throbs to the rhythm of life.

Feel your blood as it courses through your body.

Carrying oxygen and nutrients to every cell.

You are a self-contained storehouse of life.

You are a microcosm of the Universe.

You are a replica of God.

All of life pulses through you.

All knowledge is contained within you.

All can be accessed by you.

Just go within and ask, and then listen, and then feel,

and then you will know.

For all answers are within you.

For you are within ALL.

And ALL IS ONE.

The Living Library Of All Knowledge Is Located Within Each Of You.

I greet you today in the name of the One Creator of All That Is, the Living God within us all. Know that your distance from us is not far, just a few kilometers in space, and although this distance physically divides us, we are as close as the leaves are to the tree, we are as close as the wind that brushes your face, for our consciousness flows out from the depths of the Earth and reaches you to caress and bless you every moment.

We came here specifically to help this great Earth evolve and to have a home for our own evolution at the same time, and to bring you, who live on the surface, up into the higher realms of light where we can all meet and be together as One. For with our merging of consciousness we become a great force of Light that can bring all of us into higher and higher realms where all the avatars await us. So move up with us in consciousness, and flow with us through the Earth and read our thoughts on the return flow, so we can converse with one another as was meant to be; our conversing and our meeting is what will move all of us into higher dimensions of light.

We come before you this day in all our glory and splendor, bringing forth all our wisdom and cheer, to cheer you on your path, the ever winding path that never ends, that leads only upward and onward into the glory of God, the glory of God within you. For within you is ALL. All the answers you are seeking, all the explanations you need. It is all there, within your vast human temple that stores all the information of the cosmos, and we beckon you to access it.

We beckon you to follow us in thought, and as you do, we can help you resolve and solve all your earthly cares, all your earthly problems. For now that you know we're here, just call on us; we will hear you and we will respond. For this is our mission, this is our dream, to connect with each one of you on the surface, and gently lead you and guide you into the light of your higher self, the light where you actually dwell, the place where all is stored and all awaits your opening to the doors of information that lie hidden within your very being.

All life on Earth at this time has access to their inner doors of consciousness that need only be nudged to turn the lock and open. So, move these doors and open them, and you will find us here, ready to walk with you into Eternity. We are ever beaming our lights to you, we are ever beaming our love to you, and we are ever beaming our thoughts to you. Catch them, and return them to us.

We are nestled snugly in our hearths, in our homes, inside the Earth, where we are very safe and very secure, and we offer this security and this snugness to you. We offer this to you in hopes that you will follow us, and we will take you into the heart of God, which resides in your very own heart space, your very own temple of Light. We love you all very deeply. We know of your dreams and we know of your desires to live peaceful, abundant lives. So please travel with us, as we explore fully all that there is and all that you can achieve. Just know that this exploration comes from within you; you don't need to go anywhere. You can explore the depths of your very own soul and the universe from right where you're sitting. There's no need for physical travel of any kind. Just beckon to us and we will take you there. Because once you merge your consciousness with ours, we are One. And you can travel with us. We can travel together to the outermost reaches of space and to the innermost reaches of your soul. And we can unite in one consciousness and blast our way to the Stars.

The Living Library of all knowledge is located within you. From this access point within you, you have your fingertips reaching all the knowledge there is.

You don't have to physically turn the pages of a physical book; just turn the pages within your soul to rediscover all the wisdom and all the knowledge that ever was and ever will be.

You do this by going into meditation and consciously connecting with the God Source that you are, and calling on your friends in the Subterranean Cities and the Hollow Earth, your Family of Light, to be here with you and to explore the Hidden Realms with you, until the hidden realms become exposed and open pages for you to read. These are the same hidden realms that you explore nightly in your etheric body, as you leave the Earth plane and are once again free, free to be all you are meant to be. So be with us in your thoughts and explore the Hollow Earth in your visions, and see us just waiting for you to connect with us so we can take you on the journey of your life into the Hollow Globe and out to the Stars.

Synchronicity, Imagination, and Rebirth

Synchronicity Is the Result of Unity Consciousness.

This is the path that is opening to all surface dwellers. It is this path that, if you follow it, will lead you into emergence with all of us underground, and all life in the Universe.

Once you are within Unity Consciousness, all falls into place, as you are in synchronicity with all life everywhere in the Universe - not just on Earth. This is how opportunity comes to you, 'out of the blue'. Well, the 'blue' is the Universe, and once your path becomes known to 'All', 'Air is at your beck and call to arrange the instances and occurrences and resources you need to complete your mission on Earth.

It is being in the Universal flow of our Universe. This is where

We exist, as We live Underground. We are in contact with all life in our Universe, and can see and hear and feel all that occurs. This is why our lives are so magical Underground; it's not the depth of the Earth that determines this, but the width of our consciousness - and our consciousness expands with our Universe. The Universe and We are ONE.

And so are you ONE with All That Is. And as the incoming energies flow and integrate within you, your connection with life will increase, until you become fully connected - resulting in Unity Consciousness. Once this occurs, magic becomes common place, as your life absorbs the magic of being connected again to all life, everywhere. And you suddenly find yourself in God's arms - fully secure and fully protected.

This is where the intense energies, being directed to you from the Great Central Sun of our Galaxy, are taking you. They are taking you back home to the frequency you all left behind when you came to Earth. We, in the Hollow Earth, carried this frequency with Us, and because of our seclusion we were able to maintain our Unity Consciousness, and have been waiting for you to join us. Once you make this connection, all Earth goes up in flame - the Ascension Flame - and moves up into a higher dimension of evolution as quick as a wink. No time elapses between being 'there' (on the surface) and being 'here' in Unity Consciousness. So make this trip with us, for the journey will take your soul to Nirvana.

In the Hollow Earth, all we think, we create; for we are conscious of each thought and conscious of its outcome. Therefore, we can create exactly what we desire to enhance our already perfect lives. It's not 'hit' or 'miss' like it is on the surface, where you create both what you want and what you don't want, thereby bringing confusion and difficulties into your lives at the same time you're trying to perfect it - and it then seems that you are 'going nowhere'. We understand this process you go through, as we've been watching you for millennia, on our underground computer screens. You take one step forward and one step back, as you try to resolve all the difficulties and break through all the obstacles in your life.

Soon all the destructive forces will be revealed and removed from the surface, so that you are not picking up and reflecting their negativity into your lives. The veil of Maya has been pierced, and you will begin seeing the politicians and laws for what they really are — which are barriers to life, not promoters as they profess to be. We have no negative interferences in the Hollow Earth, this is why our lives mirror perfection. And soon the surface will have no negative interference, for God's energy will not integrate with negativity, and these negative entities will not survive the influx of energies which will only increase in intensity. The Earth's ascension is now assured, and your desire to live only in the Light is fully assured too. Once you cross this 'energy line', you will suddenly discover Us and all life everywhere in our Universe. It has only been the veil of maya that has caused this separation in your perception of what exists and what doesn't exist. It is your field of vision that has been blurred - for we have always been here in your time - waiting for you to put in the corrective lenses of higher consciousness that will allow you to 'see' us.

We know you as our brothers and sisters who have temporarily lost your way over the last 12 million years of surface time. Through your consciousness, you are finding your way back to who you really are, and defining the kind of life you would really want to live. The life you live now seems like freedom to your blurred vision, but as your higher consciousness focuses the 'lens of life', you are seeing that this freedom is really slavery in disguise. When you have to work long hours for basic necessities that are really free, then you are in slavery - you are chattel. The electromagnetic grids surrounding Earth can supply you with all the energy you need for free. Your governments know this, and they use it for themselves. It is their way to keep you in debt. Indebtedness is slavery, not freedom.

The longer the hours you spend daily on your jobs, the more unbalanced your lives become. It isn't the money you need, it's the time to reflect on your lives and time to spend outdoors in Nature. This is the meaning of Freedom —having the time to bring your lives to fruition, to bring your dreams into your reality, to bring your lives back into balance and to bring your families back together again into a strong framework of unity.

In the Hollow Earth, our families are in total harmony and we support one another fully in everything we do. We always have our evening meals together, and always have time to sing and dance after dinner. We really understand the term 'fun', and it is a large part of our lives.

We dictate these messages to you, to give you 'life support' from the Hollow Earth. We are your 'life support system' from Underground, and we will continue our flow of energy to you, until you have fully 'recovered' from your surface life and make the transition in consciousness to our higher realm of existence.

Your Internal Light

We are combining our light into one mighty beacon and

sending it through the crust to your surface population where it is received in their hearts.

Our life inside the Earth is always warm, sunny, and peaceful, and our spirits are always dancing with the Light of God inside. This internal reflection of the Light of God is what illuminates our minds and bodies and forms a halo of glowing light around us emanating from within.

You, too, can externally reflect your internal light. Just concentrate on your electronic current of Light energy running through your spine and magnify it through you. Know that this current connects you to the Great Central Sun, instantly electrifying you with the great Light of a thousand suns. Just see it, feel it, and know it. You are a mighty SUN. Your light alone can power all the appliances and electrical generators on Earth. This is how powerful you all are.

And once you all come into your "knowing" and "discovery" of yourself, you won't need to pay electric and heating bills, for you will provide your own internal heat and your own light, so that the elements around you adapt to your vibrational flow and raise up all life within your energy field. This is true mastership, this is the "true" you.

So focus only on the Light and Love within you, and slowly and gradually you will raise the frequency of our sweet Earth into a rising ascension tide which cannot be stopped, but will only gain momentum and velocity, and like a mighty ocean wave will crash on the beaches of the 5th dimension, spilling you all onto its shores.

Imagination Is The Real Substance Of The Universe

Greetings from Earth's interior! the silver Light, speaking to you from the Library of Porthologos, deep inside the Earth. The Light is so bright inside our home, that it shines and sparkles like silver rays of light. All our lives we've lived among riches and splendor, and wonder how it could have eluded you on the surface? If you just look around, you will see the abundance and beauty of the Earth, and yet you've failed to mirror it in your lives.

Instead you mirror the opposite of Earth's beauty. You mirror the lack and bleakness that you've created within yourselves, and think this to be the true picture of life. As your spiritual sight develops, you will begin to see the true identity of all the life that surrounds you; and then with a shocking awakening you will start out-picturing your 'real' surroundings and bring heaven to Earth. It is that simple. For heaven has always existed around you and within you, waiting for you to 'see' it.

You've created your own prison bars around your life stream, and now it is time to dissolve them with your higher vision. See right through them, and as you do, they will be obliterated by your higher sight frequency, never to return. This is how you see out into the Universe - by looking through all your past pre-conceived thoughts and beliefs and focusing on the beauty of the whole Universe; which you know is there if you can only penetrate it with your sight.

You do this through your imagination, which isn't imagination at all, but 'imaging' or focusing on what really exists around you. You've been taught that imagination is unreal - but on the contrary, imagination is very real. It is the real substance of the Universe and is how you can see all of existence while your feet still stand on Earth.

It is like 'x-ray' vision, and it is real. It is the way to see beyond ordinary sight. If you're attuned to God, you will see the beauty and truth of all existence as you concentrate your mind on it, and let it come into your imagination. For come it will, with all the beauty and splendor that you can 'imagine'. It is only your thoughts that can deplete it of its magnitude, or close it off. It is only your ancient belief system that shuts you out from the rest of existence that is teeming around you.

So open your eyes from within your imagination, and let them roam the planets and galaxy, and you will know for a certainty that 'you are not alone', anywhere you go. For life, in all its myriad forms and dimensions, is surrounding you everywhere - all attuned to different frequencies of consciousness. But you can feel the space around you, as it is charged with prana, the nutritional and energetic spark of life. Prana can free you from your dependence on food, and can fill you with its life force. All advanced civilizations on other star systems live on prana, as St. Germain does when he visits Earth in his physical body.

Prana is the substance of the Universe, and will keep your body youthful and perfectly nourished forever. As you further awaken to who you are, imagine prana flowing into your crown chakra from a tube opening and going straight through your body down into the Earth. Concentrate and 'imagine' the prana coming into you, for it will return your body to physical perfection if you can start the flow of it again and maintain it.

We, in the Hollow Earth, are nourished by prana, although we delight in eating our 'homegrown' foods too. We are healthy and strong, and never sick a day in our lives. Headaches and stress are unknown to us, for all we feel is the peace and serenity we out-picture from our surroundings.

As you rise in consciousness, you will feel more and more of the beauty and perfection of life around you, and will be able to express it through your form and feelings and thoughts until it becomes as real to you as your old self is to you now.

Spring of Rebirth

I am waiting for you in the Library of Porthologos, in the center of the Hollow Earth. We welcome you today, and are joyous to make our Sunday connection to you through the telepathic hotline. This hotline gives you access to our thoughts and our feelings, even though we are way below ground. And in the return loop, we access yours. It's a circuitous loop that connects us fully and completely as we merge our thoughts together as one.

Today it is Sunday, and as we gaze up to the stars, we feel heaven below. For heaven is where your heart is, although your body resides on Earth. April is a wonderful month of rebirth. It is the Spring of our souls, budding forth with new life and new fragrances and new hope for a new future. All life is decked out in buds and blossoms and garments of green, ready to burst forth into magnificent flowers and bushes and trees with the most fragrant of aromas. It is the turning point of the seasons, and all life waits in anticipation for this glorious event, just as all humanity waits for their consciousness to bud and bloom and open to the scent and sight and sounds of the heaven world that surrounds you. You are all prepared for a great re-birth of life, a regeneration and rejuvenation of your bodies and souls that will catapult you into the higher dimensions of life, where you will find us waiting for you. And we have waited so long. The Spring of life is finally here, and all

Earth is now blossoming into the diamond petals of the creator.

Your entry into Light has been slow and tedious, but time has speeded up, and now you are where the flow of heaven can reach into your souls and permeate your cells with the diamond light of the Creator.

A New Golden Age

My dearest residents on Earth, I am speaking to you from the Inner Chambers of the Library of Porthologos located beneath the Aegean Sea deep inside the opening in the Center of the Earth.

The Light on the surface is expanding at hyper-speed and exponentially increasing faster than we can believe. You are all in for the "ride" of your lives, racing to catch up in consciousness with your unseen brothers and sisters living inside the Earth. We can hardly wait for your masses to reach our level of consciousness, for this is when our whole Earth explodes into a Star of Great Light, and with one leap you finally reach the 5th dimension where you can see into the Hollow Earth and see us with your new eyesight. You will be so surprised at all that you see around you and up in the heavens that you never saw before.

We are so grateful to all surface dwellers for their receptivity to the Light, and for allowing the Spiritual Hierarchy to keep increasing the increments of Light to the planet. It is only with your receptivity that the Light can so intensely fill your Earth and reach your bodies. Your eons of living lives of limited consciousness are over, and your bodies are gearing for return to full consciousness. You are at the threshold of a new Golden

Age, one that is filled with only light and perfection and abundance and one that is destined to last forever.

You are the New Guardians of the Earth as the Cetaceans have passed the torch on to you - and you can finally take it and run with it in complete abandonment and joy We are your neighbors down in the Earth, but our hearts are as close to you as if we were living next door. Soon our doors will be open to you, and you can come "down" for a visit. We, in turn, will be ringing your doorbell and coming for tea. What a glorious merging of civilizations this will be. There is only hope for a future of Love and Peace - for nothing else can exist. The prophets have prophesized this time for Earth, and now it is here.

The darkness is receding and the power moguls and cabals are retreating. They have been given the order to retreat from their posts of power and control or face the consequences. They will be removed. There will be many changes in store for all the governments on Earth, as the time for the implementation of the Divine Plan for Peace is at hand.

Return of the Christ Consciousness

Hollow Earth, bringing you glad tidings for the ascension wave about to sweep the surface and funnel you into the Fifth Dimension of Light and Love and everlasting Peace. We bless you from below, as we feel the flow of energy engulfing our planet and all life in and on it.

Every living specie will be catapulted into a new world of Love and Light a world where all can continue their everlasting evolution into Eternity, free from constraint and limitations and poverty and wars.

It is "now," dear ones, the Kingdom of God is at hand, just as Jesus predicted. The return he spoke about is the return of the Christ Consciousness within your heart flame and not somewhere up in a cloud.

So stand erect, feel your sovereignty, and connect with your Holy Christ Self, bringing it fully into your physical body and experiencing the strength and understanding that surpasses all.

Feel us within you, for indeed we are a big part of you, as you are a part of us.

Your God-Selves are ready to take dominion within your hearts and minds, and this will bring your consciousness fully in union with us - where you will be able to perceive our world, even as you remain in yours. We are feeling your closeness and waiting for your consciousness to ignite with ours into one blazing light, bringing all surface humanity into the "Father's house" where there are "many mansions" that Jesus spoke of.

As you make this trip "up" in consciousness, you will also be going "down" simultaneously, enabling you to see us as clearly as you see the house across the street. You will be able to see everything that exists in your solar system and galaxy. You are so close and we are so overjoyed at your progress and your ability to absorb so much Light so quickly. We cheer you on from below and wait for the pleasure of your company. We are ready to receive you into our homes and physically embrace you in our arms. We wait and pray for your entry into our realm of Light.

Earth and Crystals

There is so much more to Crystals than what your eye perceives, for Crystals are Living Beings too. They are pure consciousness that holds memories of All That Is. They literally hold the events of the world.

Crystal energy is what vibrates the Earth, your body, and your cells. It is the vibrating force of the Universe that brings all life together as One pulse. Our pulses, and the pulses of all life forms, beat to this vibration, for it is this vibration that beats the hearts of life forms, animate and inanimate. For although we term crystals and rocks and stones as inanimate, they have a vibration that is in synchronicity with the Earth. And when we hold a crystal in our hand, it fine tunes our connection and pulse to the Earth the Mother of all life here.

Our thoughts are pulsations of energy that emanate from us in waveforms that are either in tune with our surroundings or out of tune, depending upon our vibration. Since most of Earth, at this time, is still ' out of beat", so to speak, with the forces of Nature, you can bring yourself back into the rhythm of Nature by surrounding yourselves and your homes with crystals.

Holding a crystal while you meditate is the best way to guarantee that your energy will be in harmony with the Earth. And when your energy is in harmony with the Earth, you become aligned with the Earth's magnetic grid Unes, and can access

That Is", is in perpetual flow to Earth and to yourselves, if you are tuned to her frequency.

We think this will help you understand the importance of

having crystals in your homes, and carrying them when you go outside, either around your necks or in your pockets or purses. For they emit a protective field of resonating light around you, that cannot be penetrated by anything less than this light frequency.

Crystals are much like the trees, in the respect that they, too, are waiting for you to acknowledge them as "Living Beings" encased in stone, who are ready and eager to communicate with you and become a part of your life. They have so much to offer you, as they "step up" gour vibration to levels where you are no longer feeling only the third dimensional density, ut consciousness levels where you bypass third dimension and rise to higher levels of awareness, where all life waits for your entrance so that you can finally "see and feel" beyond your physical five senses and experience the multi-dimensionality of who you, as humans, truly are.

This is how We operate inside the Earth. We are always resonating with our crystals and matching their frequency, which is why we are able to exhibit our multi-dimensionality inside the Earth because this is the only frequency we know. We always are in its crystalline flow, and we always are pulsing with our crystalline surroundings and Mother Earth's crystalline pulse rate. You, too, on the surface can match our "beat" by tuning in to us, here ui the Earth's crystalline core, and keeping crystals in your homes and pockets.

All life, everywhere, is one great flow of Crystalline Light Energy. Planets who are in this synchronized flow are of the Light, and planets who are not in this flow remain discordant and out of balance with the rest of the Universe. Earth is gradually raising her vibratory rate, and as the energy coming to you from our Great Central Sun speeds up, so does your vibratory rate, until you once again pulse with the synchronicity or our Universe. This will be one mighty pulse beat, which will move our ENTIRE Universe into a greater state of ultra-multidimensional consciousness, far surpassing its present state of consciousness, and beyond anything that anyone residing in this Universe has ever known before.

So meld yourselves with us in consciousness, as you allow your cells to resonate with ours through your imagining of us and your visions of us and your thoughts of us. These are REAL connections, although on your surface your imaginations are still considered unreal.

In reality, it is your imagination that propels you into higher states of awareness, where other life forms dwell. You can actually "see" the fairies and gnomes and elves and devas through your imagination of them, for your imagination is another one of the senses that you will soon reclaim and begin experiencing more frequently again, until you imagine or remember all that you forgot.

So beat with us in frequency, feel our hearts merged with your heart, until we are only One heart. This is how you will traverse great expanses of space, and can be with us in consciousness. It is the fastest kind of travel in existence anywhere.

Everything in the Hollow Earth

We are seated in our room in the Porthologos Library, looking out at the Stars, the Stars of heaven as they float silently by us. For even as we sit under the ground we can see out into the Universe in all directions at once. Our hearts and minds are attuned to the Creator, the Source of all Oneness and connector to all life.

We love our Earth, and as we live inside her, we are privy to all information that ever was — and to all events currently taking place on the surface as well as on other solar systems in our Galaxy. We capture, or record, these events in our Crystal Projectors, and file them away for safe keeping in our extensive library.

All our records are ancient, by your standards, as your lifetimes are so short compared to ours. But these "ancient" events existed in our lifetime since we are eons of years old in the same body, and therefore occurred during our lifetime. This gives us a different perspective of life — one that honors and reveres the Earth and all life everywhere. Because we have lived through so many ages that have taken place on the surface, we have seen and experienced the connectiveness of all life everywhere.

Which brings us back to Crystals. The evolution of Crystals is ancient also, as they have always existed and are the witness to all events on Earth. They, themselves, have recorded all the events on Earth and stored them within their crystalline network of "nerves" that can hold voluminous amounts of information.

These crystals are very evolved Beings, whose mission it is to record all that transpires on Earth, so that all that has transpired can be played back on our Crystal Projectors and learned from. For all life is a learning experience, and without the knowledge and wisdom of the past, how do you expect to learn and advance your evolution? Your books are all filled with misinformation, compiled by mankind's opinions and beliefs and theories that have little resemblance to actual conditions or facts. So all you learn doesn't give you a clue as to the real nature of Earth, the Universe, or "you".

Whenever we want to learn something and apply it to our lives, we go into the Crystal Recording Room and play back the sequence of events that will lead us to the information and wisdom we need to resolve any problem or increase our understanding of events and our lives. This is important for you, our Earth brothers and sisters; for you, too, need to have this information available to you so that you can see how your elected government officials have mismanaged the Earth's resources, and have kept you in virtual survival struggle mode for eons. Your lives are so controlled and your freedoms so diminished that you don't even know it, because it's all that you've known, and you label it democracy, equated with freedom.

How the wool has been pulled over your eyes to keep out the Light of the Universe, and imprison you on this small island floating in space! For although you can't see out, or hear the Earth calling to you, or feel the love of the trees as you scurry by them in your frantic pace of life, know that all life, everywhere, is aware of your plight and has come to your rescue to wake you up out of your deep Slumber of the Ages so that you can regain your conscious remembrance of who you are, why you are here on Earth, and the important part you play in bringing Earth out of her density and into a higher realm of Light where you will experience real "freedom", firsthand.

Your crystals can help you make this jump in consciousness, in a miniscule amount of time. Just hold them close to you, and they imprint their wisdom into your heart in "no time" at all, and raise your vibration to a place where you can readily access all the knowledge and wisdom that has been gathered throughout all time. Your crystals, no matter what size they are, can move you all into a higher state of awareness.

We, in the Hollow Earth, are surrounded by our crystals in every "walk of life" and every place we go. Our homes, transportation, work places, cultural complexes, everything is constructed of crystals and surrounded by crystals. Our buildings literally glow with Crystal Light, and our body's glow increases as we advance in our evolution. For love and wisdom and awareness IS Light and the more Light you contain within your beings, the greater the sheen of your glow.

So surround yourselves, your homes, your computers, and your work places with crystals.

Hold them and talk to them, and you will feel their consciousness being transferred to yours, and adding their Light and wisdom to yours, so that you can better access and understand the world around you, and glow like a beacon to your family and friends, who will feel the comfort of being near you — the comfort that you will radiate out to all in the radius of your energy field.

We spend so much time in our fields and forests, just basking in Nature's healing caresses, and feeling her lifestream pulsing through our veins. You, too, can feel this same pulsing of life, by spending more of your time outdoors. Now that it's Spring, you can sit and eat outdoors, as we do, instead of in your enclosed homes. This is the best relaxation there is and the best way to connect with Nature that there is by being with her and not separated from her.

The Crystals, the Earth, and all life forms are One Consciousness. When you can understand and integrate this concept of Oneness, your life will gain a new flow, and synchronicity will be a common occurrence, as you will operate on a higher wavelength that re-connects you with all life everywhere; thereby allowing you to access all the avenues that will lead you to the fulfillment of your dreams on Earth.

Know that I am always alert to your calls, and can guide you from my home underground, by your melding with my consciousness. This way, you will have double the help to guide you in your life. In fact, if you consciously stay within our frequency band, you will always find yourself exactly where you need to be, doing exactly what you need to do to accomplish your soul's purpose on Earth.

The Cetaceans communicate with each other no matter where they are in Earth's oceans, by staying in the frequency flow of "All That Is". It is the way the trees and animals and all of nature communicate. The first step is to be conscious of this interconnection of all life, and then you will find it flowing within you, with no "work" on your part. This is the key to the Universe, and it is within you.

Earth Is the Showcase of the Milky Way Galaxy

I reach out to you today, in harmony and goodwill toward all surface dwellers on Earth. We extend our friendship to you with open arms, to receive you into our lives, into our homes, and into the Inner Earth where we dwell. Harmony surrounds us all inside the depths of the Earth, and soon harmony will surround the entire Earth, as she rises in consciousness, as an ascending Star in the Heavens.

As Earth floats through space, her weary travelers climb the ascension ladder that will bring all souls into the knowingness of their beings. Due to the enormous amounts of energy being directed to Earth, a flame has been ignited in the hearts of mankind, a flame so great, that all humanity has caught the fire of God's spark of consciousness blazing in their hearts. This Light is awakening mankind to the remembrance of who they are, and the knowledge of the Universe contained in each tiny body cell.

We see the Light as it pours forth onto Sacred Mother Earth's body, igniting her atmosphere into a blazing Light that penetrates the body cells of all life on her surface. We, too, feel the intensity of this Light as it revs our vibration to speeds beyond Light. All on Earth are being blessed by the luminous Light show as Earth's aura gleams through the density that once kept her hidden in darkness.

Now her Light is seeping through the vast expanses of space, where all eyes are focused on her amazing birth into Light. She is ignited and fanned by God's Love, and all Ascended Beings, Angels, and Cetaceans carry the torch of Love that keeps her Light blazing through all lire everywhere. No one can escape her Light now. Even the darkest of souls, who refuse to budge in their positions of power and destructiveness, are feeling the Light invade their space to reveal their intent to control the Earth's populations. They love the dark, and the Light is exposing all facets of their true character for all to witness. This is creating an uncomfortable environment for them, and causing them to step up their operations and react more intensely to situations in government and politics. They will do themselves in, and bring about their own demise.

Don't get caught up in the news or the skirmishes between the Light and dark that are erupting. For they will reach a crescendo and then decline and fade away, as these souls will finally step down from their positions of power and be removed from the Earth, never to reappear again. Their time is up. And yours, dear brothers and sisters of Light, is just beginning. Soon the Earth will have a new beginning. A beginning free of coercion, where every species will thrive through Unity Consciousness, and be able to bring all their dreams to fruition. It is the dream of life, and it is soon to be the norm.

We are all in for exciting times ahead, as all knowledge that has been kept from you will be revealed. You will bask in the Light of "who you are", and remember your purpose for being here. As Unity Consciousness envelopes the Earth, she will rapidly rise in frequency to burst through the third dimensional barrier of density into the Light of the fifth dimension, carrying you all with her.

These are remarkable times, never before experienced on Earth. Soon you will be discovering hidden ancient knowledge, tablets and ancient writings that will remind you all of your heritage, and free you from life's struggle. All you need is free.

We, in the Inner Earth, are free people living free lives. And this freedom is what keeps us perpetually young in heart and young in body. For we have resolved to never deviate from God's laws. For it is God's laws that keep us in health and wealth, and that perpetuates our life spans.

All is quickening on Earth. In the Inner Realms, where all is Light and all is Love, we watch in amazement as more and more humans awaken to the call of their souls daily, and opt for peace, opt for life, opt for all that is their birthright. The Earth is the Showcase of the Milky Way Galaxy, for it is bringing all life back to the heart of God, to be reunited in one great Wave of Ascension.

We remain hidden in the Earth's core until Unity Consciousness prevails on the surface, at which time you will find us in the midst of you, guiding you and loving you and welcoming you home. I am Mikos, speaking to you from the Library of Porthologos, where I am the Head Librarian.

Confederation of Planets

We Are An Arm Of The Creator

We are part of the great brotherhood and sisterhood of Light for this part of the Milky Way Galaxy. We oversee your sector of the galaxy and solar system, and protect you from any outside intrusion intending to interfere with your evolution.

We protect you from the outlying reaches of space, where there are still pockets of dark forces that would like to overtake your planet for the wealth of resources it contains, including the human. There is a great war between the light and the dark coming to an end, and we in the Ashtar Command know with a certainty that this final battle is about to wage its last death throes leaving the earth and humans free to evolve. We watch over your skies and make sure that you are always protected as this darkness plays itself out until it just evaporates and disappears forever. We are the great forces of Light, and our cosmic assignment is to protect you always, to make sure that you regain your freedom so that you can evolve in peace and prosperity forevermore.

We are here as an arm of the Creator, maintaining peace in your sector where your solar system resides as you circle the galaxy in your everlasting trip around the sun. Soon you will be in a new position in the galaxy, one in which there is great light and brotherhood of solar systems. Where there is immediate connection of thoughts and vision, and where all are aware of each other, regardless of which planet you reside on. All work together in brotherhood of peace and love. This is what you are moving into. And this is what we are moving you toward. We will meet you there, in your new home position, where you will be able to freely and visually see and converse with us. So just look up to the sky, and visualize our star ships hovering above you and capturing you on our monitor screens. We know where each and every one of you are, always. We work together as one.

The Great Rebirthing Process

Greetings from the Space Command. I am Ashtar, your brother from the Stars, and I am with you this day of great earth activity, bringing you news of the great rebirthing process taking place on planet earth.

Unbeknownst to your physical senses, great amounts of energy are catapulting to Earth, bringing all life into greater attunement with God. Your scientists and astronomers are unaware of these events, for they base their work on outer occurrences of concrete evidence that they can gather and physically prove.

The shift that is taking place on your planet is the shift from Outer Consciousness to Inner Consciousness, away from travel to Outer Space and into travel to Inner Space. This is where the Great Exploration takes places. This is where you will find all the answers you are looking for.

Are All Planets Hollow?

Know that there's life on all the planets in your solar system.

These are your brothers and sisters living in a higher dimension than you, and whose electrons are vibrating at a greater velocity. Your electrons will soon pick up speed, and will be spinning at a rate that will propel you into the fifth dimension of Light, where we all await you.

For your information, you are all living on a HOLLOW EARTH. Your brothers and sisters who reside on other planets in your Solar System are also living on planets whose cores are Hollow. All planets in your solar system are Hollow, with life both IN and ON them.

Your sun, Helios, has a Hollow core, as all suns do. The light emanating from your sun is cold, not hot, as you have been taught to believe. It only reaches a higher temperature when it comes in contact with your atmosphere. All celestial bodies are Hollow, as this is the way they are formed. It is time that these truths were brought to earth!

We, in the Galactic Command, travel to all the planets in your Solar System, and are able to see them firsthand. Soon, you will have the capacity to travel to the other planets, and witness their true structure as well. Just know that all you've been led to believe will be open to dispute as you rise in consciousness.

Our Computer System Links Us to the Confederation

Know that the Confederation of Planets works closely with the inhabitants of the Hollow Earth and Telos. Know that we are in constant communication with them through our Computer Systems. Know that we monitor the whole Earth surface and below the surface.

Someday soon, you will have access to this vast computer

system that's based on amino acids, and you will be able to plug into our vast monitoring network in the Cosmos. Then you will have the information and guidance you will need to stay in a state of balance and harmony with the Earth. This is all waiting for you, waiting for the energies to bring you and all life forms into the necessary state of consciousness that will allow us to implement this grand plan of bringing forth to you our vast computer system that will network you to the Stars.

We Trees Are The Ground Crew

We trees are here in service to the Ashtar Command, too. Only we are the "ground crew" who have "dug in" and live in our "dugouts," so to speak, while doing the same job and having the same assignments as you, who walk on foot and travel on land. It's just that our "physicality" is stationed in one spot, while our leaves blow hither and yon in the wind, and our scent and voices travel far inland.

For we communicate with all living life on the surface, just as you do. Our boughs reach through many dimensions as we stand guard on earth, and we are privy to information coming in on different wavebands also. Our auras are vast and connect us to one another across space, and we span Earth's globe and hold her tightly within our auric arms of green and gold. We bless the earth, for she has given us life, life to reveal our innermost natures and life to express ourselves in myriad of ways and forms.

For as you walk, we talk, and our voices ever follow your footsteps, guiding you on your path through nature's innermost realms where you can play and experience the magic of our species, albeit, in different forms.

This is 'My Tree' in my backyard who channels messages to me, and when I sit under her branches, she becomes an extension of me, and is my antenna to the stars.

Ascension

Earth is Shifting into Higher Dimensions

We have only your highest good in mind. All we think is the goodness we feel in our hearts for all of humanity. Your Earth is shifting into the higher dimensions at a rapid pace, and your loss of time is your confirmation of this shift. Notice how quickly your days pass. Disregard the negativity you read about and hear on the news. It is the last stand of the dark forces, as they rear their heads in one last battle to dominate the Earth. Their time is over. A new Earth is dawning, a new sun is rising, and a new heaven is at hand. A glorious time is approaching. It is the freedom you all dream of, being birthed into your present.

In the Hollow Earth, heaven is all we experience, and if there were clouds we would 'walk on them' as your saying goes. Soon, you too, will feel the exuberance of 'walking on clouds', as your clouds literally fade away and your atmosphere 'lightens' up as the density dissolves and the pollution decreases, to bring your clarity of mind into focus as the new heaven descends upon your Earth plane and you, at last, can touch the stars.

So much is happening at levels you are not consciously aware of yet, to bring you all fully into the Light and back into the Confederation of Planets.

Earth has not been lost. On the contrary, its been saved by the

Lightworkers who are emitting more and more Light daily, and the company of heaven who have dedicated their lives to raising Earth into the higher vibrations.

All Life Forms are Opting for the Ascension

All life forms presently on Earth are opting for the ascension. However, some will ascend with the Earth and with us at this time, and the others who have been unconscious of their inner choices and unwilling to ascend at this time, will do so at a later time. Know that the Earth's ascension is assured, and that we will all be moving our location closer to Helios, our Sun.

The people in the Hollow Earth are overjoyed with the rise in frequency that has taken place over the last few years. We yearn to connect with you in the physical, and now this connection is fully assured. We can even "guarantee" this, as you would say above. Yes, you are above us, but depth of location is irrelevant. For with peace coming to the planet, all life will be assured of rapid evolvement to make up for the lost days of darkness.

Humanity has learned its lesson well, and has learned the futility of war and bickering, and cries now for an end to the insanity. And the end is coming. You are witnessing the last eruptions on the surface.

From this point on, you will begin to see the merging of peoples, places and principles, as all come together in ONE UNITED EARTH. This is the day God has been waiting for. This is the day your holy God Selves have been praying for. This is the day we will open up the tunnel exits and come to you, with our brightly colored robes and sparkling sandals, bearing gifts of immense riches and the necessary devices that will return your planet to its pristine state once again, for we can solve all your pollution and sickness problems in just moments.

Timelines for Earth's Ascension

Today we will speak about the timelines for Earth's Ascension. Know that there are vast amounts of Light flowing to Earth from the Great Central Sun and beyond, including all Universes in our multi-universe system. All systems, everywhere, are aware of what is now occurring on Earth, and all are sending their support in the form of light waves. All these light waves are converging onto Earth's atmosphere and funneling into every cell of every life form on Earth, including our Earth herself. This is a spectacular revelation for beings on Earth to comprehend, and a spectacular sight to witness. All density is being lifted, felt, and dissipated into the ethers forever transmuted to light, never to return anywhere again.

As all this is occurring, you are imperceptively being lifted higher and higher into the light frequency that you left when you came to Earth. Your bodies are being renewed and regenerated at a level you do not physically feel, and yet it is occurring moment by moment until such a frequency is reached that you will suddenly explode into the diamond light that you are. It is all about reaching critical mass and timelines. The timelines for all this to occur, are closing in on your Earth, and converging from every direction and dimension, until they all close in upon one another and explode into now. And then you are there! There with Us in consciousness, and there with all life, located everywhere in all universes simultaneously.

What an event to be able to witness, let alone be a part of as you all are. This has never been done before, anywhere in all existence. This is why there are vast numbers of beings from great numbers of universes here, circling your Earth, watching all this happen, and waiting for the great moment of synthesis to occur. And when it does, there will be great rejoicing throughout all the multiverses and beyond.

It's all about timelines and consciousness reaching a critical mass, and then everything takes off exponentially at a speed beyond anything you could conceive. The speed happens at a now moment, with no time elapsing at all. Ah, the wonders of God's creation.

Wait out the remaining timeline patiently, knowing that all will come to a glorious conclusion of instantaneous awakening for all life on Earth, jettisoning you all up to the stars, and down to us, of course.

Solar Flares

Today we will talk about how you are being bombarded by solar flares from your sun. This is all in anticipation of the new day dawning on Earth, the new day when all life will be free.

The solar flares are burning away the negativity that is concentrated in the hearts of mankind, so that your heart energy can finally be freed to rise to connect you to your god Selves that wait patiently just a few feet above your heads. This is all part of the Divine Plan to free humanity from the grips of darkness that have enshrouded your Earth for eons. So look to your sun as your savior, for its light is purifying your planet as it gives you its warmth.

Critical Mass

Today it is calm in the Hollow Earth, as it is on all days, except for this special day of Sunday, as we wait for you to take our dictation. On these Sundays, there is a special breeze in the air, a breeze of anticipation as we connect with you again. It is as if the whole Hollow Earth stirs, knowing that it is time for us to deliver our dictation to you. It is a knowingness that pervades our air and we are all aware of it. So here you sit, with all our energies surrounding you, as you take our dictations. Our whole library knows of these Sunday channelings, and everyone sends their love to you. You are so surrounded by our love. Our hearts are connected to yours, and we are ready to begin.

Greetings from the Library of Porthologos. Today the flowers are in mighty blooms of reds and purples, and their scents are wafting through our nostrils with the most delicious of fragrances. We pass these fragrances on to you, and hope you can capture their scents as you sit above us at your computer. We bring you good tidings and blessings of love from all the people in the Hollow Earth. More and more of us here below, are connecting with more and more of you above. It is indeed a wondrous time, in which all the prophecies are about to be fulfilled in this 7* golden age on earth. All of humanity are desiring peace, and people are waking up now by the thousands. There are now over 29 million surface humans awakening to who they are, and the critical mass that we are hoping to reach before 2012 is 55 million.

With this critical mass achieved, we are assured of the 10,000 years of peace. It is also this critical mass that allows the Ascended Masters to visibly and physically walk the Earth surface, to openly teach the Universal Laws to mankind. So there are great changes ahead, and the changes all point to peace.

We in the Hollow Earth are pleased beyond anything we can

express. For all these humans awakening, points to our soon being able to emerge from our homes beneath the Earth, and physically join with the Lightworkers on the surface, where we too, will be teaching humanity the Universal Laws of life. All life on Earth is preparing to ascend, and help is coming from planets and star systems of which you don't even know exist. When people start questioning, and asking themselves the universal question of "who am I", then it is a sign of awakening, a sign that their soul is longing to know, longing to remember again. And once this question is asked, even though it is just a whisper, this gives the Ascended Host the opportunity to step in directly and begin teaching on a conscious level. But until people ask this profound question, we cannot directly help them. And once this question is asked, the whole universe jumps in to respond, and this person is added to the Tist' of awakening ones.

Know that we in the Hollow Earth know everything that transpires on the surface. We know the results of your presidential elections, and we are amazed at how the American people were so easily deceived and lied to, and how little they questioned the election process.

Our love for surface humanity goes deep, and we wish we could be on the surface now, giving our love and support to those lightworkers who are in need of us. For down here, we don't ever work or live alone, we always have our circle of friends, or groups, that we work with.

These groups are our main support systems, and we work and travel together. This is what is lacking on the surface. Your families are all splintered and separated, and you have lost your group support system, which is crucial to life. Imagine the joy and fun of working on projects together, and receiving constant support?

Our love to you pours forth from the center of the Earth, and spirals into your heart in blazing colors of the rainbow. As you sit at your computer, you can feel these heightened sensations of contact, just as we can feel yours. It's this stepping up in vibration that happens whenever we connect in consciousness. It is our dream to someday be sitting right here in this room next to you, planning our workshops and talks to the populace. The best way to reach people is by working together, and we look forward to working with you as soon as we are on the surface.

Quickening the Soul

Our journey here is almost over, as the Light descends on you, our surface brothers and sisters, gradually bringing you all up to our frequency. When your light quotient reaches our frequency in intensity we shall all instantaneously merge into ONE GREAT LIGHT from both above and below. It is at that instant that you will see us, as we emerge from our hidden homes underground. We are ready for this; it is the Quickening you've all been waiting for, and that Jesus talked about. It is the quickening of your souls to the Light - to quickly integrate the Light into your very own cells so that you shine as a beacon on Earth.

All life everywhere in the Universe of Alpha and Omega, is waiting for this quickening to occur. It occurs by opening your heart flame to all life on Earth, especially those within your relationships. As this Light expands in you, it lights those you're connected to, and leaps as a hot ember from your cells to others in your proximity, thus igniting their cells simultaneously and expanding their Light. It is as if you were all standing in one gigantic bon-fire of light, and watching the flames as they flow into you and then out to everyone you come in contact with, including Mother Earth. It is a gigantic bon-fire of life, and you are throwing off sparks in all directions - just like fireworks; only these sparks catch and hold and integrate and expand, quickening the soul who is receptive to it.

Earth is creating quite a stirring in the Universe, for this time ALL of Earth will be ascending, igniting the 'domino effect' which will catapult this whole galaxy into the higher dimensions. It is the glory of God rejoicing. It is the Stars exploding, and it is your heart expanding into the One Heart of Creation.

Love Is The Key

Blessings my Sister above. It is Mikos, your brother from below, beginning this two-way session with you. Today we will talk about Love - Love for humanity that all people from below hold in their hearts for all people above. Yes, we hold immense, infinite Love in our hearts for all humanity living above ground. This is one of the purposes of our being here, to hold this love and constantly direct it to surface humans, so that the spark never goes out, but expands and expands until it ignites the spark within each of your hearts and explodes into the divine flame fully encompassing your beings with the light of the sun, that in that instant, brings you home to the heart of Creation.

All is love and all is light and all awaits your return journey home. Home is where the heart is - and the heart is the home of God - the eternal light of Creation.

Here in the Hollow Earth, our love is a stream of light that we send forth to quench your thirst and bathe your soul, until you yourselves can emit this light and connect it to ours. Once this occurs, all Earth will go up in a flame, and ascension of all will occur. This can happen just as easily now as it can later. For love is the key As you learn to unconditionally love yourselves and love others, your lives naturally evolve, with no effort involved. Love is the base. And from love, all goodness is created. It is the alchemists secret that turns everything you touch into gold. So stretch your hearts to encompass all the love we send your way, and in turn shower your loved ones with it so that it spreads through your families and friends and workplaces. Become a 'love shower' everywhere you go, knowing that you are giving God's love wherever you are. You are here now as messengers of God, carrying God's message of love and hope to all mankind. You are the Christ returned, you are the Second Coming. It is you, not we, who bravely volunteered for this Earth assignment to bring love and light back to the surface. You are the spiritual warriors here to eternally free Earth from the clutches of dimensional density, and release her into the current of Light that will return her to the spiral of evolution where she can climb upwards through Eternity, instead of being stuck in the same rut as she has for the past 12 million years.

We are so eager for you to join us, for your hearts are pure and we 'see' that you truly want only peace and wellness in your lives. Your calls go out to the Universe, where all of God's creation responds by sending love back to you.

Reunion

A Swift Journey in Consciousness Your Journey Home

Greetings from the Library of Porthologos, inside the Hollow Earth Realm of love and light, peace and abundance unlimited. I am Mikos, and gathered around me are my fellow brothers and sisters, anchoring the energy for this channeling session. We are all so very excited whenever we meet for these sessions, for these sessions are the only avenue we presently have to get our messages up to the surface for dissemination. So we love you and bless you for your service to Earth in relaying our thoughts. For our thoughts carry the love vibration we have for the people of Earth, and our eagerness to assist you with the ascension process through our words of wisdom and guidance.

We are here to guide you in your inward journey home. The trip is all within and, therefore, free of expenses and free of travel arrangements. You just sit quietly, focus on Us inside the Hollow Earth, and we will guide you to discover the gems within your own soul. We will help you mine the resources of your Being so you may discover the wealth that dwells within you. So start your inward journey now. know that you have hooked onto our vibration, and we are fully aware of you. Call to us now as we know your frequency and will embrace you in our love. We will work with you from below, whenever you call to us from above. The words in this book automatically attune you to us, and from this attunement we become aware of your desire to be with us in consciousness. And through our intermingling consciousness, we will guide you on your journey home. We will work with all who call to us. When we make this heart connection, it solidifies our partnership to work together on the Inner Planes and to offer you the guidance you need to make your jump in consciousness. Once this jump is made, you will find us here, where we have always been, only then you will be able to see us, and you will see that we've always been beside you, had you been able to look far enough.

Drama in Optical Illusion

We send you greetings of love from beneath your soil, which is our rooftop. You are residing on the roof of your home, rather than inside. It's as if you build a house, climb a ladder to its roof, and set up housekeeping. You will soon become aware of other planets in the Milky Way Galaxy, and see for yourself the humans residing on the inside of their home planets, leaving the outside surfaces barren and free. You will be taking this visual trip as your visual acuity sharpens and your optic nerve opens and responds to the rising energy coming to Earth. Grand visions are awaiting you all, as our solar system and galaxy are responding to increased incremerits of Light and Love pouring forth from the Great Central Sun of Suns, from Alpha and Omega, the Creators of our Milky Way Galaxy. Your vision will be unlimited - all density and veils will fall away, and you will see life in all creation as it is and not through the dense optical illusions you now experience. The veils are even now being removed from the corneas of your eyes, by ever increasing light waves emanating from the Great, Great Central Sun. You will dance yourself into ecstasy as your vision unfolds and the stars and planets come into your sight and you focus and move into them as if they were just a stone's throw away - as indeed they are — only your vision has been blocked by your negative programming and illusion of being separate and apart, rather than connected and intertwined with all life in existence.

My, you are in for a great surprise! And we in the Hollow Earth can hardly wait to see the look on your faces as we make eye contact with you from our inner depths to your outer surface, and watch you blink in amazement as you look back into our eyes and laugh in excitement as you realize we were here the whole time and you just didn't see us. What a wondrous time is in store for us all, as we all finally connect and merge our consciousness into one.

It is all over. Beloveds. The struggling and pain are over. It was never meant to be. And as deep as you fell, your rise will be rapid, and you will make up the time lost, and excel in your evolutionary journey and raise your level of consciousness to great heights in only moments.

The script is already written; you are now just playing out your parts. But as the "drama" quickens, you gain momentum and carry the act to its divine conclusion with a "stand-up" audience applauding and cheering your bravery and stamina in the longest drama in illusion ever enacted. The curtain closes and you return home. It has ended.

We wait to receive you in our homes of crystal and gold, and treat you to our sumptuous meals and walk hand-in-hand with you through the Hollow Earth, treating you as the Queens and Kings, Goddesses and Gods that you are. We await your visit.

Message to Dianne

You are a direct descendent of us and have chosen to incarnate on the surface to bring our two worlds together. We are the Inner Earth Beings, and we are working directly with you and many others on the surface. We are imparting our knowledge of existence to you on a subconscious level, where you will have direct access to it as your vibratory rate increases. We will converse with you whenever you call on us.

We understand your yearnings and desire to be in contact with us, but know that you spend much time here in your dream state. You walk among us, and converse freely with our people while your body rests in your bed. You are attending our centers of Higher Learning. We are working with you in your sleep state, and consider you our representative on the surface.

Our lives are tranquil and peaceful, and this tranquility gives us the opportunity to evolve rapidly, and to delve into whatever sources of study we wish to learn. This is the purpose of life - to ever evolve in an environment where all have access to the myriad wonders of the universe.

Know that we keep our Inner Earth safe, and are vigilant and caring individuals. We regret the monstrosities that are occurring on the surface, and we lament the state of affairs and horrendous acts of killings in the Middle East and elsewhere. If we were to intervene directly, what could we do, and who would listen to us? We could come to your aid, but only the Lightworkers would accept us, and the rest of humanity would turn against us. Therefore, we remain underground, just as the Telosians remain underground at this time. We are hoping to come to your aid at the time of the great merging of our many civilizations in the different strata of Earth. Only God knows this timing, and the Spiritual Hierarchy guides us all unerringly.

We remain your brothers and sisters even though you have little contact with us, much less than you've had with the subterranean cities. They are the advance guard, so to speak, with us following. So stand guard over your Earth, and maintain your Light and center of gravity at all times, then nothing will blow you away from your mission to reunite all of Earth's peoples.

We are the group consciousness of the Inner Earth Beings, and we love you and admire your tenacity to endure the above conditions. Blessings, our brothers and sisters.

Crossing Over Dimensions

Our lives are so totally free compared to yours. We fly, while you crawl. You are all blessed to be on Earth at this time, as this is the crucial crossing over of dimensions leading to a new world of Light and Love for Earth. All of life is anticipating this crossover, and millions of Beings from other worlds are here witnessing it. You are all going on this journey together.

There will be no further interference in the evolution of humankind, thus giving everyone the opportunity to ascend in the minimum of time necessary. Your Earth has asked the Spiritual Hierarchy to speed up the process of evolution so that all can begin a swift journey in consciousness.

How to Connect with Us

Greetings, our Brothers and Sisters of Light. We reside inside your precious Earth, ever ready to communicate with you. We have been here for hundreds of thousands of years, waiting for this glorious day to appear, when we could begin our communications with you on a regular basis. The time frame is now. All, whose intent is pure, can now connect with us through your heart flame, for we have the same flame in our heart as you do. It is the one flame of the Creator's divine spark of life. We are all connected through our heart flames, lighting up the world by our linkage. As we turn our connections on with each other, our auras become generators and transmit our light out into the universe where all can see it. We exponentially light up our whole Earth. This is what our oneness does - it lights up the Earth, carrying it to a higher level of consciousness which, in turn, moves us all higher up the ladder of evolution until we are catapulted into the next dimension where we will find ourselves automatically linked to everyone and everything. Our heart's connection is the key that opens up the universe and lets us in. And once in, we are forever united in consciousness as ONE. So as you connect to us, you connect to everyone, everywhere, through us.

We Have Established a Link in Your Area of New York

We are gathered around you now, sending you our Love and our deepest longings for reunion with you and surface folk. We have established this link with you in your area of New York, to connect us with your part of the country. We have done the same in other locations, so that when the time for our emergence comes, we will have specific persons in specific locations that we can 'physically' contact. This is most important at this time, as our emergence becomes more and more possible as each week passes. So we humbly thank you for meeting with us each Sunday, as this link strengthens our connection with each channeling session. We leave you for now, and will continue our dialogue next Sunday. We send you our Love, and bolster your heart with our energies through the week between our channeling.

Earth's Glorious Future

We are meant to live in joy, and learn only from joy. Many of you on planet Earth at this moment are Starseeds and not originally from Earth. You have volunteered to incarnate as Earthlings many times so you can be prepared for this final time. You are members of the "Family of Light". You are here to firmly anchor Light onto the planet. Your work is honored by so many Beings in the Universe, that you will wear the colors of gratitude for eons to come.

The colors of your Auric Field will say "I Was There". No matter where you travel in the Universe, you will be flocked by Entities wanting to find out how it was done. How did you lift the Earth out of the darkness and turn her into a Star. For the next two thousand years, she will be the brightest Star in the Milky Way. Her Goddess Essence will illuminate our part of the Universe. Her rays of Light will carry the language of Love the one true emotion of creation. She will become the main hub for our Galaxy. She will become a Living Library that will attract Beings from the outer reaches of the Universe who are seeking knowledge in order to enhance their evolution knowledge that can only be accessed by the Human experience.

Every experience is unique, but the Human experience holds the keys to ancient information of many Star Nations that worked together to seed the Earth with the best their civilizations had to offer. Hence the saying 'every human is perfect'.

In the past, many Galactic civilizations had given up on her. But not the Family of Light. They knew deep within their souls that Earth was a gem they could not afford to lose. So they swung into action and devised a plan that was so brilliant it even caught the attention of Prime Creator. You are on Universal television. And the ratings have become so high that millions of civilizations have put their evolution on hold to see the final episode.

So stick around, because after the final episode we are throwing a party of Galactic proportions. Every Being that has ever walked on planet Earth will be there. And if you think that we from the Hollow Earth look different, just wait till you see what's coming. Forever, Mikos and friends."

Addendum

Its citizens are survivors of the sinking of the Lemurian continent that occurred about 12,000 years ago. Their isolation from the surface population has enabled them to create a civilization of peace and abundance, with no sickness, aging, or death. The word 'telos' means "communication with spirit." Telos is one of over 120 Cities of Light that are only a few miles beneath the Earth's surface. As a grouping, these are called the ' Agartha Network.'

About the City of Telos

We are human and physical just like you, except for the fact that our mass consciousness holds thoughts of only Immortality and Perfect Health. Therefore, we can live hundreds and even thousands of years in the same body.

We came here from Lemuria over 12,000 years ago, before a thermonuclear war took place that destroyed the Earth's surface. We faced such hardships and calamities above ground that we decided to continue our evolution underground. We appealed to the Spiritual Hierarchy of the planet for permission to renovate the already existing cavern inside Mt. Shasta, and prepare it for the time when we would need to evacuate our homes above ground.

When the war was to begin, we were warned by the Spiritual Hierarchy to begin our evacuation to this underground cavern by going through the vast tunnel system that's spread throughout the planet. We had hoped to save all our Lemurian people, but there was only time to save 25,000 souls. The remainder of our race perished in the blast.

For the past 12,000 years, we have been able to rapidly evolve in consciousness, due to our isolation from the marauding bands of extraterrestrials and other hostile races that prey on the surface population. The surface population has been experiencing great leaps of consciousness, in preparation for humanity to move through the Photon Belt. It is for this reason that we have begun to contact surface dwellers to make our existence known. For in order for the

Earth and humanity to continue to ascend in consciousness, the whole planet must be united and merged into ONE Light from below and ONE Light from above.

It is for this reason that we are contacting you; to make you aware of our underground existence so you can bring the fact of our existence to the attention of our fellow brothers and sisters above ground. Our book of channeled messages from Telos is written to humanity in hopes that they will recognize and receive us when we emerge from our homes beneath the ground, and merge with them on the surface in the not too distant future. We will be grateful to you for the part you play in helping us broadcast the reality of our existence.

Secrets of the Subterranean Cities by Juliette Sweet

The Agartha Network

Think of Shamballa the Lesser as the United Nations of over 100 subterranean cities that form the Agartha Network. It is, indeed, the seat of government for the Inner World. While Shamballa the Lesser is an inner continent, its satellite colonies are smaller enclosed ecosystems located just beneath the Earth' s crust or discreetly within mountains. All cities in the Agartha Network are physical, and are of the light, meaning that they are benevolent spiritually based societies who follow the Christie teachings of the Order of Melchizedek. Quite simply, they continue in the tradition of the great mystery schools of the surface, honoring such beings as Jesus/Sananda, Buddha, Isis and Osiris. . . all of the Ascended Masters that we of the surface know and love, in addition to spiritual teachers of their own longstanding heritage.

Why did they choose to live underground? Consider the magnitude of the geological Earth changes that have swept the surface over the past 100,000 years. Consider the lengthy Atlantis and Lemurian war and the power of thermonuclear weaponry that eventually sunk and destroyed these two highly advanced civilizations. The Sahara, the Gobi, the Australian Outback and the deserts of the U.S. are but a few examples of the devastation that resulted. The sub-cities were created as refuges for the people and as safe havens for sacred records, teachings and technologies that were cherished by these ancient cultures.

Spotlight on Telos

How can over a million people make their home inside Mt. Shasta? While we're stretching our imaginations, our neighbors, the Japanese, have already blueprinted underground cities in answer to their surface area problem. Sub-city habitation has, for thousands of years, been a natural vehicle for human evolution. Now, here is a peek at a well-thought-out ecosystem.

The dimensions of this domed city are approximately 1.5 miles wide by 2 miles deep. Telos is comprised of 5 levels.

LEVEL 1: This top level is the center of commerce, education and administration. The pyramid-shaped temple is the central structure and has a capacity of 50,000. Surrounding it are government buildings, the equivalent of a courthouse that promotes an enlightened judicial system, halls of records, arts and entertainment facilities, a hotel for visiting foreign emissaries, a palace which houses the "Ra and Rana Mu" (the reigning King and Queen of the royal Lemurian lineage,) a communications tower, a spaceport, schools, food and clothing dispatches and most residences.

LEVEL 2: A manufacturing center as well as a residential level. Houses are circular in shape and dust-free because of it. Like surface living, housing for singles, couples and extended families is the norm.

LEVELS3: Hydroponic gardens. Highly advanced hydroponic technology feeds the entire city, with some to spare for intercity commerce. All crops yield larger and tastier fruits, veggies and soy products that make for a varied and fun diet for Telosians. Now completely vegetarian, the Agartha Cities have taken meat substitutes to new heights.

LEVEL 4: More hydroponic gardens, more manufacturing and some natural park areas.

LEVEL 5: The nature level. Set about a mile beneath surface ground level, this area is a large natural environment. It serves as a habitat for a wide variety of animals, including those many extinct on the surface. All species have been bred in a non-violent atmosphere, and those that might be carnivorous on the surface now enjoy soy steaks and human interaction. Here you can romp with a Saber-Toothed Tiger with wild abandon. Together with the other plant levels, enough oxygen is produced to sustain the biosphere.

LANGUAGE: While dialects vary from city to city, "Solar a Maru," translated as the "Solar Language," is commonly spoken. This is the root language for our sacred languages such as Sanskrit and Hebrew.

GOVERNMENT: A Council of Twelve, six men and six women, together with the Ra and Rana Mu, do collective problem solving and serve as guides and guardians of the people. Positions of royalty, such as are held by the Ra and Rana Mu, are regarded as ones of responsibility in upholding God' s divine plan. The High Priest, an Ascended Master named Adama, is also an official representative.

COMPUTERS: The Agarthean computer system is amino-acid based and serves a vast array of functions. All of the sub-cities are linked by this highly spiritualized information network.

The system monitors inter-city and galactic communication, while, simultaneously, serving the needs of the individual at home. It can, for instance, report your body's vitamin or mineral deficiencies or, when necessary, convey pertinent information from the akashic records for personal growth.

MONEY: Non-existent. All inhabitants' basic needs are taken care of. Luxuries are exchanged via a sophisticated barter system.

TRANSPORTATION: Moving sidewalks, inter-level elevators and electromagnetic sleds resembling our snowmobiles within the city. For travel between cities, residents take "the Tube," an electromagnetic subway system capable of speeds up to 3,000 m.p.h. Yes, Agartheans are well versed in intergalactic etiquette and are members of the Confederation of Planets. Space travel has been perfected, as has the ability for interdimensional shifts that render these ships undetectable.

ENTERTAINMENT: Theatre, concerts and a wide variety of the arts. Also, for you Trekkies, the Holodecks. Program your favorite movie or chapter in Earth history and become a part of it!

CHILD BIRTH: A painless three months, not nine. A very sacred process whereby, upon conception, a woman will go to the temple for three days, immediately welcoming the child with beautiful music, thoughts and imagery. Water birthing in the company of both parents is standard.

HEIGHT: Due to cultural differences, average heights of subterranean citizens vary — generally 6'5" to 7'5" in Telos, while nearly 12' in Shamballa the Lesser.

AGE: Unlimited. Death by degeneration is simply not a reality in Telos. Most Agartheans choose to look an age between 30 and 40 and stay there, while, technically, they may be thousands of years old. By not believing in death, this society is not limited by it. Upon completing a desired experience, one can disincarnate at will.

ASCENSION: Absolutely, and much easier and more common than on the surface. Ascension is the ultimate goal of temple training. Why have they stayed underground all this time? In part, because the Agartheans have learned the futility of war and violence and are patiently waiting for us to draw the same conclusion.

They are such gentle folk that even our judgemental thoughts are physically harmful to them. Secrecy has been their protection. Until now the truth of their existence has been veiled by Spirit. When can we visit? Our entrance to the sub-cities depends on the purity of our intentions and our capacity to think positively. A warm welcome from both worlds is the ideal and must be expressed by more than just the lightworking community.

Currently, a few hundred brave subterraneans are working on the surface. In order to blend with the masses, they have undergone temporary cellular change so that, physically, they don't tower above the rest of us. They may be recognized by their gentle, sensitive nature and somewhat mysterious accent. We wish to introduce you to Princess Sharula Aurora Dux, the daughter of the Ra and Rana Mu of Telos. Sharula has been officially appointed Ambassador to the surface world by the Agartha Network. She was born in 1725, and looks 30. This article is courtesy of her firsthand experience.

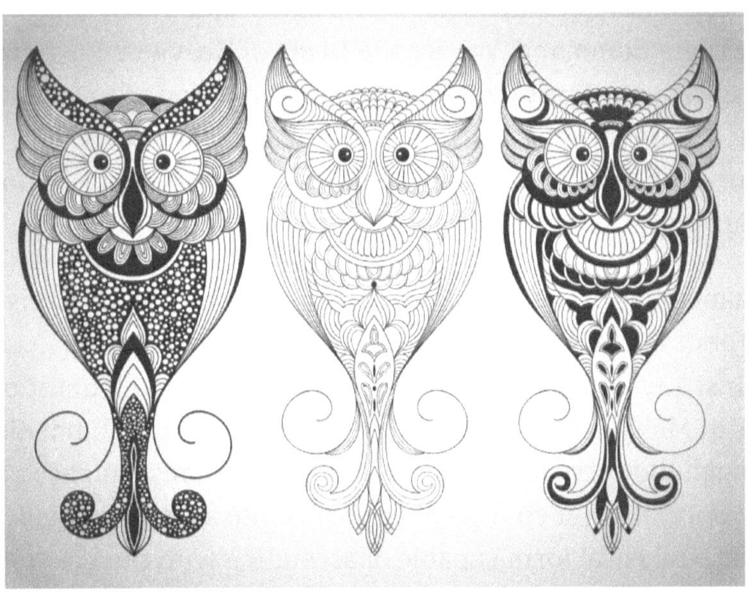

THE ASHTAR GALACTIC COMMAND

THE ASHTAR COMMAND is the airborne division of the Great Brother/ Sisterhood of Light, under the administrative direction of Commander Ashtar and the Spiritual guidance and directorship of Lord Sananda Kumara known to Earth as Jesus Christ our Commander-in-Chief. We are also known as the Galactic Command, the Solar Cross Fleets and the Orion Jerusalem Command. We are the Hosts of Heaven who serve the Christ, our Most Radiant One, in His mission of universal love. We can best be understood as celestial or angelic in nature, functioning as councils of Light upon missions of Holy endeavor in accordance with the Divine plan.

As a member of the Galactic Confederation. we oversee this sector of the Milky Way Galaxy protecting the Divine plan against any type of interference or violation of confederation Law or Melchizedek protocol. We are here to assist humanity through the current dimensional shifting in consciousness, the transformation of your physical forms into a less densified etheric-physical form capable of ascending with the Earth into the fifth dimension. We also work in coordination with our brothers and sisters in Telos and their Earth based Silver Fleets under Commander Anton and with the Melchizedek High Priest of Telos, Adama. We are all working together under the authority of the Office of the Christ, the Great Central Sun Hierarchy (Throne of God), and the Order of Melchizedek. We also have our bases located within mountain ranges, in desert areas and under the oceans. We, our bases and our Merkabahs (aerial chariots or starships), are invisible unless we wish otherwise. In order to see us your vibration would have to match the wavelength upon which we are manifesting. We, and our higher dimensional vehicles are composed of etheric matter, as real and solid to us as your environment is to you. Thus we appear by lowering our wavelength to match the third dimensional vibration and we disappear by raising our vibrations beyond your visibility range.

We would like you to know that you are not alone in the universe nor anywhere else for that matter. What you do affects not only your world but countless other civilizations and worlds existing in different dimensions but just as desirous of maintaining their existence as you are yours. In fact, Ashtars first personal entry into your solar system occurred in 1952 in response to urgent reports that Earth was attempting to detonate the hydrogen atom, a living organism, an act in violation of Confederation law. The state of the pollution and decline of your planet's ecosystem as well as your delving into nuclear fission for defense purposes caused him to immediately send delegations from the High Council of the Ashtar Command to meet with certain heads of your planetary government. We do all that is possible without violation of your free will to neutralize excess radiation within your soil and atmosphere and to deflect potentially dangerous asteroids from impacting your planet.

We maintain the stability of your planetary axis and as much as possible relieve the pressure of your tectonic plate systems thus directing earthquake activity away from heavily populated cities. We constantly monitor all geophysical and astrophysical conditions affecting Earth as well as other planetary systems. We are universal ambassadors of peace, peacemaker/ diplomats and peacekeepers, and we greatly anticipate the day when you too will join us within the United Federation of Peaceful Worlds.

The Ashtar Command is composed of thousands of starships and millions of personnel from many civilizations. We also have many members of the Command currently living on Earth, some having been born into Earth families, and others who come and go, living for a time amongst their brothers and sisters on Earth and then returning to their respective points of cosmic origin.

Life upon Earth and throughout this solar system was originally seeded by the Elohim, so it is very similar if not identical in form. We are all Rays of the one God-Source-Creator and as such have the Divine duty and mission to extend God's love throughout all time and space continuums. It is you who give a face, voice and hands to God's love in your world. You are in the End Times, the last days of war, conflict and harmful intent. Sooner than you can possibly fathom, you and your precious orb will move into a kinder, gentler version of your world. It has simply outworn peaceless existence as a viable or allowable option. Within less than twenty years the Earth and all upon her will transform into a world of pure love. Those not willing or capable of making that transformative adjustment will find themselves in the world of their choosing.

The Divine Plan is always perfect and always just. Watch for the miracles occurring daily in your life and worldwide. These will continue until you realize that you are deeply loved and part of a plan more beautiful and wondrous than you could have ever imagined. We are sending you messages of love and universal truth via crop circles, designs ever more intricate and exquisite. We are even sending circles and cross patterns of light to adorn your buildings and glow in your windowpanes.

Please stop a moment and contemplate how you live and move and have your being within such a great God! Know that you are an embodiment of Divinity designed to be fully indwelt by the Holy Spirit. That is your real nature and calling in life and you will only find genuine and lasting joy and peace when you give unconditional expression to the love that you are. Ask, it will be quickened within you. Please also receive our love that we offer to each one of you upon your beautiful planet.

You may know us as your elder brothers and sisters, as the coworkers of Christ upon a mutual mission of love. We are the celestial heralds of the good news of God's love for all of His Creation and of the entering of your world into a higher dimension of understanding, revelation and life more abundant. In the Light of our Most Radiant One we bid you God's Blessings.

THE SMOKY GOD

The Smoky God is the real life account of a Norwegian sailor named Olaf Jansen. His story, set in the 1800s, is told in Willis Emerson's biography entitled: "The Smoky God." Olaf's little sloop drifted so far north by storm that he actually sailed into a polar entrance and lived for two years with one of the colonies of the Agartha Network, called "Shamballa the Lesser." He describes his hosts as those of the central seat of government for the inner continent . . . measuring a full 12 feet in height . . . extending courtesies and showing kindness . . . laughing heartily when they had to improvise chairs for my father and I to sit in. Olaf tells of a "smoky" Inner Sun, a world comprised of three-fourths land and one-fourth water.

"During his Arctic flight of 1,700 miles BEYOND the North Pole he reported by radio that he saw below him, not ice and snow, but land areas consisting of mountains, forests, green vegetation, lakes and rivers, and in the underbrush saw a strange animal resembling the mammoth..."

"For years rumors have persisted that on his historic flight to the North Pole, Admiral Byrd flew beyond the Pole into an opening leading inside the Earth. Here he met with advanced beings who had a sobering message for him to deliver to mankind on the Surface World."

"Upon Byrd's return to Washington, on March 11, 1947, he was interviewed intently by top security forces and a medical team. Our government branded him as a lunatic and kept him drugged and locked in an asylum in the interest of national security."

Here, from Admiral Byrd's secret log and diary, is the message meant to have been heard 56 years ago!

Excerpt from A Flight to the Land Beyond the North Pole:

"I bid you welcome to our domain, Admiral." I see a man with delicate features and with the etching of years upon his face.

He is seated at a long table. He motions me to sit down in one of the chairs. After 1 am seated, he places his fingertips together and smiles. He speaks softly again, and conveys the following: "We have let you enter here because you are of noble character and well-known on the Surface World, Admiral." "Surface World," I half-gasp under my breath! "Yes," the Master replies with a smile, "you are in the domain of the Arianni, the Inner World of the Earth. We shall not long delay your mission, and you will be safely escorted back to the surface and for a distance beyond. But now. Admiral, I shall tell you why you have been summoned here. Our interest rightly begins just after your race exploded the first atomic bombs over Hiroshima and Nagasaki, Japan. It was at that alarming time we sent our flying machines, the 'Flugelrads,' to your surface world to investigate what your race had done. That is, of course, past history now, my dear Admiral, but I must continue on. You see, we have never interfered before in your race's wars and barbarity, but now we must, for you have learned to tamper with a certain power that is not for man, namely, that of atomic energy. Our emissaries have already delivered messages to the powers of your world, and yet they do not heed. Now you have been chosen to be witness here that our world does exist. You see, our culture and science is many thousands of years beyond your race. Admiral." I interrupted, "But what does this have to do with me. Sir?"

The master's eyes seemed to penetrate deeply into my mind, and after studying me for a few moments he replied: "Your race has now reached the point of no return, for there are those among you who would destroy your very world rather than relinquish their power as they know it..."

I nodded, and the Master continued. "In 1945 and afterward,

we tried to contact your race, but our efforts were met with hostility. Our Flugelrads were fired upon, yes, even pursued with malice and animosity by your fighter planes. So, now, I say to you, my son, there is a great storm gathering in your world, a black fury that will not spend itself for many years. There will be no answer in your armies; there will be no safety in your science. It may rage on until every flower of your culture is trampled and all human things are leveled in vast chaos."

"Your recent war was only a prelude of what is yet to come for your race. We here see it more clearly with each hour... do you say I am mistaken?"

"No," I answered, "it happened once before, when the Dark Ages came and they lasted for more than five hundred years." "Yes, my son," replied the Master, "the Dark Ages that will come now for your race will cover the Earth like a pall, but I believe that some of your race will live through the storm; beyond that, I cannot say. We see at a great distance a new world stirring from the ruins of your race, seeking its lost and legendary treasures, and they will be here, my son, safe in our keeping. When that time arrives, we shall come forward again to help revive your culture and your race.

Perhaps, by then, you will have learned the futility of war and its strife...and after that time, certain of your culture and science will be returned for your race to begin anew. You, my son, are to return to the Surface World with this message..."

With those closing words, our meeting seemed at an end. I stood for a moment as in a dream... but, yet, I knew this was reality, and for some strange reason I bowed slightly, either out of respect or humility, I do not know which.

Suddenly, I was again aware that the two beautiful hosts who had brought me here were again at my side. "This way. Admiral," motioned one. I turned once more before leaving and looked back toward the Master. A gentle smile was etched on his delicate ancient face. "Farewell, my son," he spoke, then he gestured with a lovely, slender hand a motion of peace and our meeting was truly ended.

Quickly, we walked back through the great door of the Master's chamber and once again entered into the elevator. The door slid silently downward and we were at once going upward. One of my hosts spoke again, "We must now make haste. Admiral, as the Master desires to delay you no longer on your schedule timetable and you must return with his message to your race."

TELOS

The Call Goes Out From The Hollow Earth And The Underground Cities.

Telos is an ancient Lemurian City of Light that is real and exists to this day in the physical realm, underneath Mt. Shasta. Meet Adama, the High Priest of Telos, as he describes the kind of Earthly paradise they have forged for themselves as they raised their consciousness to let go of all violence and negativity. Because they have moved into a consciousness of total love and true Brotherhood, it has been possible for them to survive from the time of the sinking of the continent of Lemuria until now. They have created Heaven on Earth for themselves in their Subterranean Cities and throughout the Hollow Earth. They are looking forward to coming out, when we are ready, to teach us how to do the same here on the surface.

This book is a must for those of you who are seeking your ancient roots and heritage. This book will open your mind and heart to the great possibilities and wonders that are awaiting us, on the surface, when we finally let go of the old paradigm of duality and discord, and turn to Love and true Brotherhood for all. This book brings all of us so much hope for a better and easier life here on this planet.

Explore the rich family life of the people from the lost continent of Lemuria, who have been subterranean for the past 12,000 years; and who, due to their isolation from the surface population, have created a civilization of peace and abundance, with no sickness, aging or death.

Read about the Advanced Civilizations that live in peace and brotherhood in the Center of our Earth, which is Hollow, and contains numerous physical cities of Light, its own Inner Central Sun, with oceans and mountains still in their pristine state. Vividly and heroically, Telos delivers a clear understanding of what is required on the surface to create a prosperous society and a healthy environment. The Telosians and other spiritually advanced civilizations do indeed exist inside the Earth, and they are coming forward at this time to inspire us to follow in their footsteps.

The Call Goes Out:

Messages from the Earth's Cetaceans Interspecies Communication Dianne has been a telepathic channel for the Cetaceans in previous incarnations, and channels the ONE GROUP MIND of the Cetaceans. Since early on, she has been connected to the Cetaceans, and was an active member of

Green Peace in the seventies.

In a personal message to Dianne, they expressed the following: "We are the Cetaceans, awake also at this early Earth hour, floating along with the currents and sending our love to all on Earth in their sleep state. We breathe the clean air as it comes in off the shore, where humanity hasn't yet polluted it with exhaust fumes from their automobiles and factories. These early hours are the sweetest and the cleanest time to breathe deeply, for the vigor of God deeply permeates the air at these early hours. Keep you heart space open to our transmissions; for although our species differ in form, in consciousness we are one".

"We are here in our full consciousness, waiting patiently for Earth's children to bloom into the Caretakers you were meant to be. Your DNA was tampered with by past civilizations and by renegades from Outer Space. This has slowed down your evolution to the point where up to now you were barely crawling. With the huge input of energy being directed to your Earth within the last few years, your evolution is again picking up speed, and you will soon blast off into full consciousness, and will at last be with us in the higher dimensions."

This work of attunement is also a call for help. Help required for the waste that is dumped into the oceans, for the melting of the polar caps due to air pollution, for destruction of the Rain Forests, and for our need to listen to the Earth and hear her messages. Indeed, the reader will find the insightful words of Keiko, Star of the Free Willy movies; Corky, an Orca Whale incarcerated in Sea World, San Diego, California; and Lolita, an Orca Whale, imprisoned in the Sea Aquarium in Miami, Florida, among others.

DISCOVER QUANTUM HEALTH THERAPY

There is an actual place within you, where the frequencies of life are so precisely tuned and harmonized that time stands still and perfect health exists. Science has identified that place as "Quantum." It is not a fairy tale - it is a real place. It is the place where the Son and God coexist in unified Oneness. Jesus called this place, Father's House and you can only enter into "The Garden of Spirit Oneness" as a consciously awakened Spirit-Person.

Science has developed a computer that communicates interactively with you through Quantum Therapy technology. It activates and synchronizes the harmonics in your inner Spirit self to restore a healthy atmosphere within your Spirit Life Body. From my own experience, this is a true statement. During numerous sessions I have witnessed quantum therapy bring relief to those suffering ill health by synchronizing their bodies' frequencies with the harmonics of the Perfect Heart. The cost of quantum therapy is far far less than a doctor visit or hospital stay. Because it is Quantum, the therapy can be accomplished wherever you are located, without the need for personal physical contact. For example, the cell phone technology has advanced to the point where now there are billions of people who each have a personal frequency (their own individual cell phone number) which allows them to communicate with others around the world without physical contact. Likewise, the quantum computer, tuned to the unique frequency of your own heart, can synchronize your body's harmonics to a healthy state.

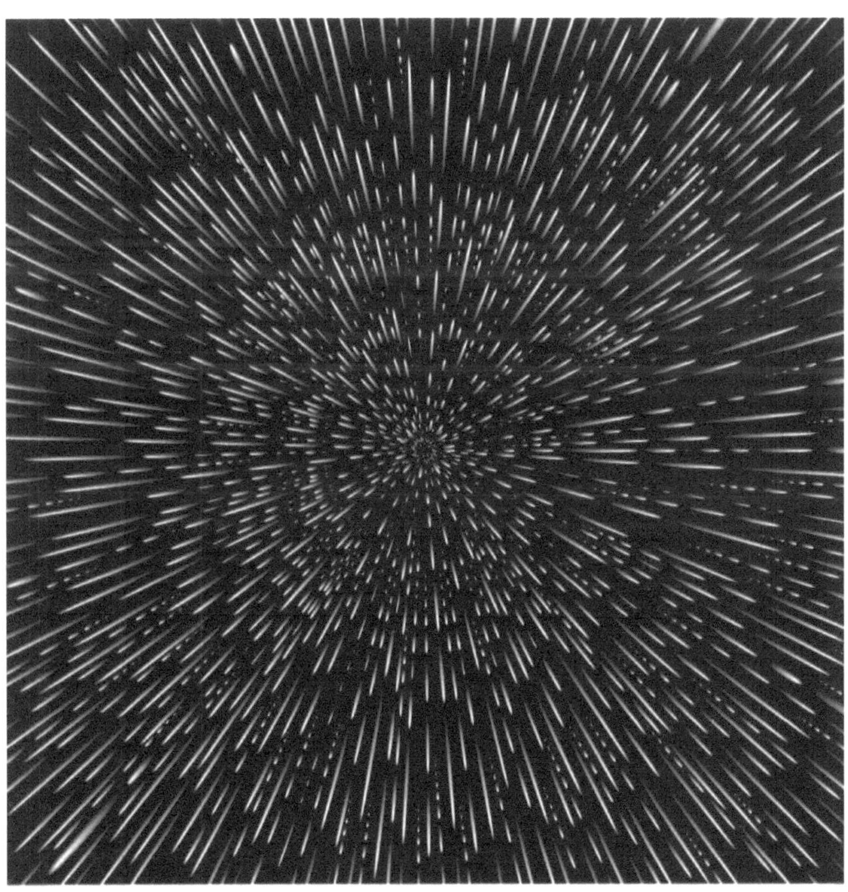

THE POWER OF QUANTUM HEALING

The Age of Aquarius has given mankind the new paradigm of the Laws of Quantum Physics.

These laws are a gift to us from the Grand Architect of the Universe, the Prime Mover, the Creator God.

They are meant for all humanity, not just for a select few, how think they have the right and privilege to know the Universes Secrets.

The New Laws of Quantum Physics are the Laws of Creation. And when we, the ordinary people, fully understand them we will understand that there are no secrets of the Universe.

We will understand that there are no secrets to physical atoms, protons, quanta or any of the theories for the physical Universe. The Physical Universe only exists as a physical object because we exist to experience it.

What are we? Well we are not physical beings, we are spiral

energy beings. To be more precise, we are Souls.

We 'blinked out' of what the Laws of Quantum Physics call the Quantum Ocean, which in reality is the Mind of The Creator God.

There are not secrets when you understand that there exists an infinite ocean of thinking, intelligent energy called the Quantum Ocean, Mind of God.

This Mind of God, is an infinite Soul. We live, move and have our being within this infinite Soul.

We 'blinked out' into a physical reality, an individual incarnation for one reason only, to experience physical Life. When we 'blinked out' this physical reality we experience, 'blinked out' with us.

Each Soul 'blinks out' into it's own physical reality. There are as many physical realities in the planet as there are Souls on the planet.

But if no Souls 'blinked out' then there would be no physical reality of any kind.

So 'physicalness' does not exist unless there is a Soul who can experience and observe it.

Spiritual Quantum Physics is just that. Only the term Quantum refers to the smallest unit of Spirituality, which is an individual soul.

And an individual Soul is just one drop in the infinite ocean called the Quantum Ocean. Spiritual Quantum Physics gives us a new paradigm for health.

It tells us that we are individual Souls who have 'blinked out' of the Quantum Ocean, mind of God, to experience "Life" on the physical, emotional, mental plane.

To do this, each Soul builds a physical, emotional and mental body to use to "Experience Life."

Within the Quantum Ocean, Mind of God, there are an infinites number of Divine blueprints that can be 'blinked out' into the physical reality to be observed and used by individual Souls.

There are Divine Blueprints for planets, Galaxies, and even Universes. There are Divine Blueprints for the Mineral Kingdom, the Plant Kingdom, and the Animal Kingdom.

And there is a divine blueprint for man, within the Divine Blueprint for man, are Divine blueprints for perfect physical, mental and emotional health.

The one big difference between the Kingdom of Man and the other kingdoms, is that we have been given free will.

We, as individual Souls, have 'blinked in' and 'blinked out' of the Mind of God many times.

Each time we do, we bring back to the Quantum Ocean, with us, our experiences, conscious and unconscious. We set up our Karma with which we will take out into the physical world with us next time we 'blink out.' Even negative thoughts, negative feelings, negative actions are also energy.

But they are energies that interfere with energies, which creates perfect health on the physical plane.

If each Soul would incarnate out of the Quantum Ocean, Mind

of God, with no negative energies, they would 'blink out' with a perfect health matrix.

And they could experience Life with Perfect Health.

But this is not the case nowadays. Mankind has drifted so far from the concepts of Spiritual Quantum Physics, IE ALL IS ENERGY, thoughts and things and we are not physical bodies, with Souls. We are Souls who create our own physical bodies.

The great thinkers, teachers, doctors, religious leaders have created a world of materialism where physical bodies are more important than SOULS.

One-by-one, we must get back to Spiritual - Quantum - Physics.

One-by-one we must understand that we are Souls, Spiritual Beings creating our own physical realities.

One-by-one we must understand that any illness we have are caused because we are thinking or feeling negative thoughts. Or we are accepting and attracting, the negative thoughts and feeling around us.

The greatest minds, physical scientists, doctors, professors, who start with the basic premise that 2+2=5 (involving No Creator God) are wrong.

They cannot find the secrets of the Universe, God or even perfect health by dissecting the physical Universe. But that is what they are doing.

The physical universe does not exist outside of the Quantum Ocean, Mind of God unless at least one Soul exists there to experience it and observe it.

Thoughts are things and each Soul creates their physical reality by what thoughts they think and what thoughts of others they choose to believe.

If this is true, then the powerful thoughts of a physicist, a scientist and a doctor create what they are thinking.

If a physicist is thinking about black holes, a scientist thinking about Atomic Bombs and doctor thinking about diseases, what do you think they are in turn CREATING?

One-by-one let us not accept their thoughts or their physical reality.

Let us continuously create our own physical reality.

Let us spend time daily thinking that we are individual Souls who live, move and have our bing within an infinite Soul, called the Creator God.

Let us spend time daily thinking that within this infinite Soul there is a Divine Blueprint for perfect health that we can attract into our physical reality by thinking about it.

A great teacher 2000 years ago, said at the beginning of the Age of Pisces: "Come ye out from amongst them. Let the Dead bury the Dead."

Now at the Dawn of the New Age, the Age of Aquarius, and the new paradigm of Spiritual Quantum Physics that saying rings truer than ever.

Come ye out from those who think 2+2=5. No matter who many college degrees they have. The physical reality you are experiencing all around you is your mental creation.

Constantly think 2+2=4, Spiritual Quantum Physics. Remember what you think and believe now will also affect your next 'blink out". What you THINK you BECOME.

Ragnar Storyteller (AKA Ellis Peterson is a Korean War Vet living with his wife Lory and dog Dixie in the boonies of the Pocono Mountains. He is a retired math professor and electronics engineer. He has written over 200 articles and booklets on runes, radionics, quantum physics, viking history, orgone generators and alternate healing methods. Ragnar is 70+ but looks 50's thanks to his inventions.

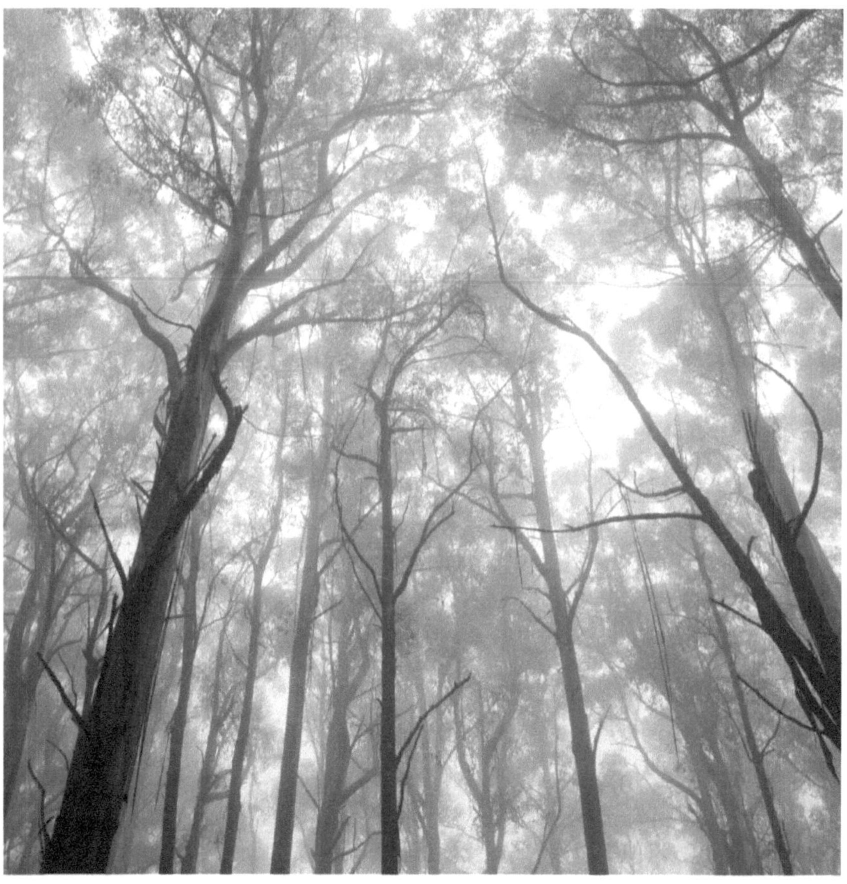

QUANTUM PHYSICS AND HEALTH MIND OF GOD

The Mind of God

We have just moved into the 21st Century and the Age of Aquarius. It is time to drop all the old Age of Piscesian (the last 2000 years) ideas of dogmatic religion and health. We are no longer in the Age of Pisces (I Believe) where we must accept the belief system and ideas of anyone else.

We are in the Age of Aquarius (I Know) where we can have direct experiences in matters of religion and health. It is no longer necessary for us to have a middle man. The biggest lie perpetuated by the materialistic scientists of the past age is the 'Big Bang Theory.' They would rather perpetuate the 'belief' that the planet Earth has come about through a hap-hazzard CHAOS. They have completely left out the Creator God, having a Divine Blueprint, or PLAN for the evolution of planet Earth, our Solar system, and our Universe.

For the next 2000 years we must bring the concept of a Creator

God back into our lives. The Creator God or the 'Big G,' who far surpasses any religious concepts which we may have held up until now, created this wonderful ever expanding, ALIVE, Universe that we live in. He/She has also put all the wisdom and knowledge of the past, present and the future into an infinite ocean of thinking, intelligent energy called the Quantum Ocean, which is the Mind of God itself.

We are also given the Laws of Quantum Physics, resonant frequencies and attraction. We can now use these laws to attract better health for ourselves and our loved ones. Within the Quantum Ocean, Mind of God, are the Divine Blueprints of all perfectly creathed things. The Divine Blueprint for man is there. The Divine Blueprint for all animals, plants, insects and minerals are there.

The Divine Blueprint for man's perfect health is there. But down through the Ages man though his ignorance has built false infrastructures over this Divine Blueprint for perfect health that we carry around within us. It is our individual, personal energies caused by our wrong thoughts, emotions and actions, (as well as the mass mind we are connected to), that has built this pattern of ill-health around us.

The Creator God has built the pattern or Blueprint for Divine Health and placed it in the Quantum Ocean for us. We can attract this Divine Blueprint for perfect health out of the Quantum Ocean, Mind of God, into our Aura, energy field. Once this Divine Blueprint of perfect health takes hold in our Aura, it will start to dissolve all the negative thoughts and emotions that reside there. Soon it will completely over ride our old health patterns with the New Divine Health Pattern.

Nobody knows how long this will take, It depends on the

individual. Each of us have different mental and emotional blockages to be worked through. Know that the Creator God, like a Knowing Creator, wants you to have perfect health. Know that God has placed a pattern or Blueprint for perfect health in the Quantum Ocean. Know that God has given us the Laws of the Quantum Physics to bring out of the Quantum Ocean what we need. Know that all creation is simple and that man has complicated it. Know that if you practice this simple following exercise, faithfully and daily you will attract this Divine Blueprint for health into your life.

Let us begin. Sit comfortably in your favorite chair, relax and breathe slowly and deeply. Now intone mentally: "I am now inhaling the Divine Blueprint for perfect health, out of the Quantum Ocean, Mind of God into every cell of my body."

Take a deep breath. Feel every cell in your body being invigorated and changed with this new energy. Do this three times. Now get up and go about your daily business, knowing that the Laws of Quantum Physics are now attracting perfect health out of the Quantum Ocean, Mind of God into your body.

Patience! It is the Creator God's Law. It WILL WORK!

Ellis Peterson AKA Ragnar Storyteller is a retired math professor and electronics engineer. He has been studying astrology, runes, metaphysics and alternate healing treatments for over 30 years. He is 70+, in very good health and lives in the boonies of the Pocono mountains with his wife Lory. His writings are unique and refreshing.

QUANTUM LAW OF ATTRACTION TIMING

We are now starting our 2000 year journey into the Age of Aquarius. With this new age comes a new paradigm called the Laws of Quantum Physics. There are two schools of thought pertaining to these new Quantum Laws. One is the school championed by the Universities, mathematicians and physicists. They are searching for truth and meaning to life in the laboratories and the classroom. Then there is the school of Spiritual Quantum Physics. This is the one I choose to write and talk about for several reasons.

One, it includes a Creator God, a grand architect, who put the whole Universe in motion, who put all the energy in the Big Bang Theory in the first place. Who placed you, I and the Universe under Natural Law. Who wants us to have a better life.

I reject the God of Chaos and the Big Bang Theory.

Besides, what good is the new paradigm of the Laws of Quantum Physics for the common folk, if it is locked up in the

Universities to be used and studied by a select few.

The age of the select few is over. The Age of Aquarius has torn the lid off the box of secrets. It is the select few religious leaders, politicians, professors, lawyers, doctors and CEO's who have help create the mess we are in. There is no room in the New Age of Aquarius for them. They will become as extinct as the Do Do birds.

So, I say let us use the new paradigm of the Laws of Quantum Physics for answers in OUR every day life. The most popular of the new laws is the Law of Attraction. This law tells us that what we think about, we attract and what we attract creates our life. The major problem with many who use the Law of Attraction for health, wealth and love is the timing factor. To explain this Quantum Timing factor, we must go back to basics.

First of all, the Laws of Quantum Physics tell us that there exists an infinite ocean of intelligent energy called the Quantum Ocean. There is no time nor space there. Everything that is was or will be exists there. It is a timeless, space-less infinite point where you, I and the Universe exist.

It is the Mind of the Creator God.

Now you and I 'blinked out' of the Mind of God as individual souls, onto the physical plane. We 'blink out' to experience "Life." And to use the experience to fulfill our destiny, This is the destiny of all souls who have 'blinked out.' And that destiny is to evolve, become more conscious, individualize and become more God-like.

We are a soul that builds a physical body, and emotional body, as well as a mental body. We are not a body who has a soul. We are a soul who has a body. The connecting link between us, as individual souls, and the Quantum Ocean, Mind of God is our Aura. Simply speaking, what ever energies we carry in our Auras uses the Law of Attraction to create our lives.

Our present health, wealth, and happiness is a direct result of the energies we carry with us. The energies we carry in our Auras we have put there with our thoughts. But understand this also. Much of our ill health and poverty and unhappiness has also been put into our minds by others.

Thoughts are things and if we want to change our state of health, wealth and happiness we must change our thought. Also we must learn to guard ourselves from the negative thoughts of others. Using our thoughts we can attract better health wealth and love out of the Quantum Ocean into our Auras. But here is the catch that many do not understand about the Law of Attraction.

Our Auras are already full. And if we are poor, sickly or unhappy or feel unloved, our Auras are full of these negative energies. The new healthier, wealthier, loving energies we are thinking out of the Quantum Ocean, Mind of God, cannot instantly enter our Auras and manifest as health, wealth and love. Quantum Time is needed. The time it will take these new positive energies to work their way through and dissolve the negative energies we have been carrying around in our Aura.

For some it will be like the slow drip of pure, clean water drip, drip, dripping into a 55 gallon drum of dirty water (your Aura.) For some it will be like a steady stream of pure clear water flowing from a tap into a 55 gallon drum.

IN CONCLUSION

Balance throughout the human body is what we seek to sustain in holistic health.

Be healthy! Heal yourself now by making positive experiences in every way you can. Quantum healing will not only improve your health condition but will heal your whole being. Let the healing energy flow and experience the benefits of good health.

Health is not found in a miracle pill, it is a way of life. Nutrition rebuilds and regenerates tissue without poisoning some other part of the body. The right biochemical elements accelerate health and the reversal process.

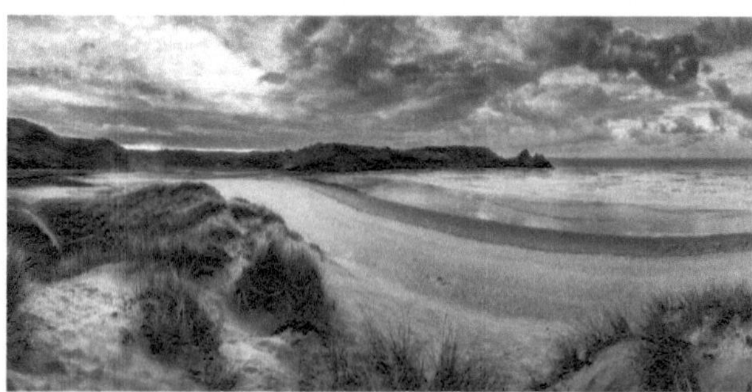

REFERENCES:

The Way to Shambhala, Edwin Bernbaum, Anchor Books; 1st edition,

Sherwood Fox, Greek and Roman Mythology

Mircea Eliade, Zalmoxis, the vanishing God: comparative studies in the religions and folklore of Dacia and Eastern Europe,

Myth: its meaning and functions in ancient and other cultures

John A MacCulloch, Celtic Mythology, Rowman & Littlefield Pub Inc

T. Write, Saint Patrick's Purgatory: A medieval Pilgrimage in Ireland

Harold Bayley, Archaic England: An Essay in Deciphering Prehistory from Megalithic Monuments, 1919 Online Edition: Link

Philip Freund, Myths of Creation

George, Wally – Pilgrimage To The Devil., Article in Fate magazine, Aug. 1957

Clark B Firestone and Ruth Hambidge, The Coasts of Ilusion, Harper & Bros; First Edition, 1924

Martha Warren Beckwith, Mandan-Hidatsa myths and ceremonies, G. E. Stechert, 1937

William Martin Beauchamp, Iroquois folk lore: gathered from the Six Nations of New York, I. J. Friedman, 1965

Pages from Hopi history, Harry Clebourne James, University of Arizona Press

Arizona and the West, Volume 17, University of Arizona Press

Harold Osbourne, South American Mythology. New York: Peter Bedrick Books

Halley, Edmond, An Account of the cause of the Change of the Variation of the Magnetic Needle; with an Hypothesis of the Structure of the Internal Parts of the Earth, Philosophical Transactions of Royal Society of London

Halley, Edmond, An Account of the Late Surprizing Appearance of the Lights Seen in the Air, on the Sixth of March Last; With an Attempt to Explain the Principal Phaenomena thereof;, Philosophical Transactions of Royal Society of London,

Ferdynand Ossendowski (1922). Beasts, Men and Gods. New York: E. P. Dutton & Company.

George & Helen Papashvily, – Anything Can Happen., Harper & Bros., New York, NY., 1940

Cave of the Ancients, Lobsang Rampa, Random House, 1993

There are Giants in the Earth, Michael Grumley, Panther Books

Peter Kolosimo, Not of this World, Sphere Books 1974 ISBN 0-7221-5309-0 also see Peter Kolosimo, Timeless Earth, Citadel Pr, 1988 Edition ISBN 0-8065-1070-6

Walter Kafton-Minkel Subterranean Worlds: 100,000 Years of Dragons, Dwarfs, the Dead, Lost Races and Ufos from Inside the Earth Loompanics Unlimited

Alien races and Fantastic Civilizations., Serge Hutin, Berkeley Medallion Books, 1975. In the Bowels of the Earth: Refers to the mysterious catacombs beneath Paris, and other underground mysteries which lead inside the Earth.

The Under-People, Eric Norman, Award Books, 1969

Inner Earth People And Outer Space People, William L. Blessing, Inner Light Publications, 2008 Edition ISBN 1-60611-036-5

Chinese ghouls and goblins, G Willoughby-Meade, Stokes co, 1929

Mysteries of Ancient South America, Harold T. Wilkins, Citadel Press., New York, 1956

"Fantastically Wrong: The Legendary Scientist Who Swore Our Planet Is Hollow | WIRED". wired.com. Retrieved 1 November 2015.

Yenne, William (2003). "Adolf Hitler and the Concave Earth Cult". Secret Weapons of World War II: The Techno-Military Breakthroughs That Changed History. New York: Berkley Books. pp. 271–72. ISBN 0425189929.

Abdelkader, M. (1983). "A Geocosmos: Mapping Outer Space Into a Hollow Earth". Speculations in Science & Technology

Notices of the American Mathematical Society, (Oct. 1981 and Feb. 1982).

On the Wild Side (1992), Martin Gardner

On the Wild Side, 1992, Martin Gardner.

Seaborn, Captain Adam. Symzonia; Voyage of Discovery. J. Seymour, 1820.

Lewis, David. The Incredible Cities of Inner Earth. Science Research Publishing House, 1979.

Kafton-Minkel, Walter. Subterranean Worlds. Loompanics Unlimited

Standish, David. Hollow Earth : the Long and Curious History of Imagining Strange Lands, Fantastical Creatures, Advanced Civilizations, and Marvelous Machines Below the Earth's Surface. Da Capo Press

Lamprecht, Jan. Hollow Planets: A Feasibility Study of Possible Hollow Worlds Grave Distraction Publications.

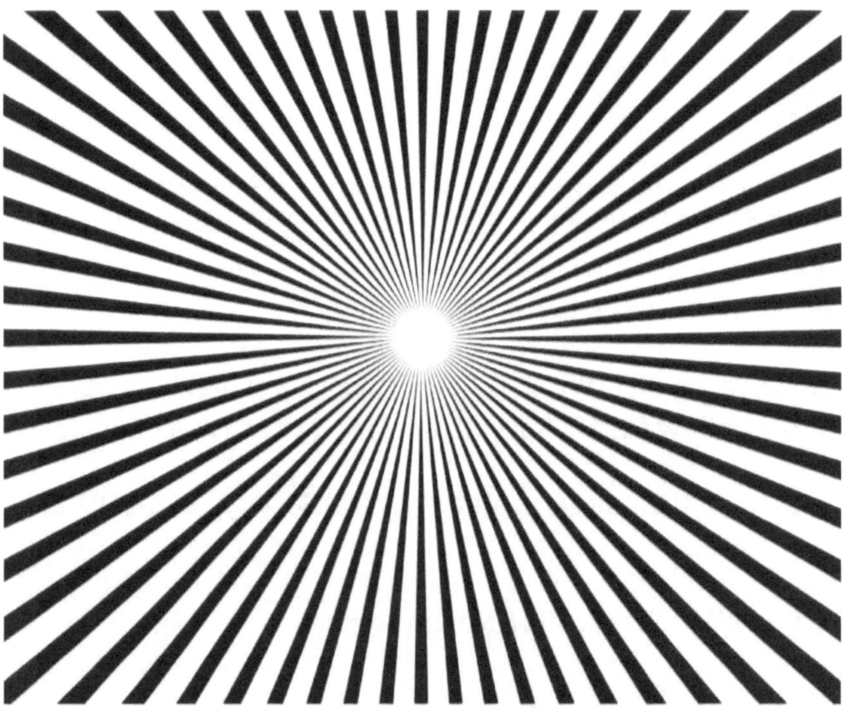

ABOUT THE AUTHOR

Dedicated to natural law, Dustin Lee Den Hood enjoys writing the truth about nature, aging, and health and how they are all connected. When he is not writing, he can be found spending quality time with family, hiking in the mountains with his beloved and his dogs, and researching natural ways to improve health and decrease aging. He lives in Alberta, Canada, with his family.

My Website is

https://QuantumHealthHQ.shop

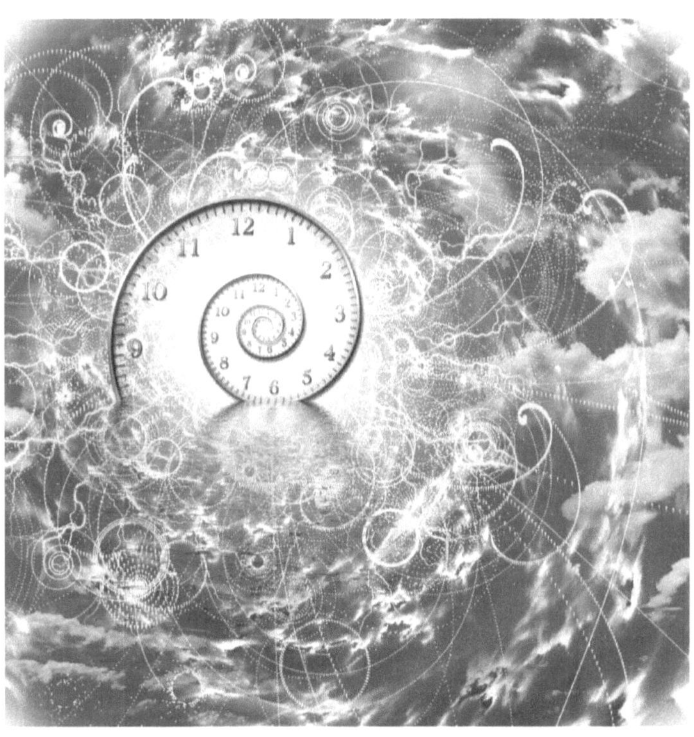